THE COMPLETE AROMATHERAPY GUIDEBOOK

A Comprehensive Reference of the Natural Holistic Healing Powers of Essential Oils for Your Mind, Body, Spirit... and Comfort Zones

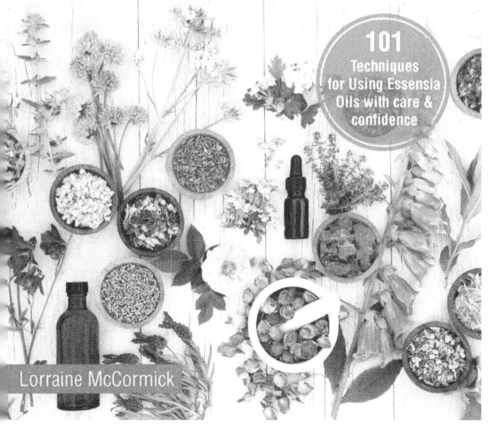

101 Techniques for Using Essensia Oils with care & confidence

Lorraine McCormick

The Complete Aromatherapy Guidebook

*A Comprehensive Reference
of the Holistic Natural Healing Powers
of Essential Oils
for the Mind, Body, Spirit...and Comfort Zones*

Lorraine McCormick
© October 2018

TABLE OF CONTENTS

Introduction 8
BOOK—I 16
Essentials Of Essential Oils 16
Chapter 1 - Aromatherapy: An Abstract 16

    Detailed Definitions 17
    Recorded Roots & Anecdotal Accounts 20
    Concept and Context 27

        Appropriate Administration 28
        Constituent Composition 30
        Product Potencies 32

    Bonuses & Benefits 33

Chapter 2 - Art of Aromatherapy: Abiding Advised Approaches 50

    Production Processes 50
    Blending Basics 61

        Concocting Combination Calisthenics 64
        Essential Oil vs Carrier Oil 70
        Dilution Do's and Don'ts: 74

    Safekeeping & Storage 76
    Safety Standards 80
    Procurement Practices 85

        Purchasing Parameters 85
        Pegged Prices 89

    Tools of the Trade 90

        Essential Equipment for Blending Basics 92

Chapter 3 - Nature's Nourishments 95

    Fragrant Flowers | Healthy Herbs: Aromatherapy Aromas 96

        1-Allspice 96
        2-Ambrette Seed 97
        3-Angelica 98
        4-Anise 99
        5-Arnica 100
        6-Balm (Lemon) 100

7-Balsam (Canadian) 102
8-Balsam (Copaiba) 102
9-Balsam (Peru) 103
10-Basil 104
11-Bay Laurel 105
12-Bay (West Indian) 106
13. Benzoin 107
14-Bergamot 108
15-Birch (White) 109
16-Boronia (Sydney Rose) 110
17-Cade (Cajeput) 111
18-Calamintha 112
19-Camphor (White) 112
20-Caraway 113
21-Cardamom 114
22-Carrot Seed 115
23-Cascarilla 116
24-Cassie 117
25-Cedarwood (Atlas) 117
26-Cedarwood (Texas, Mexican Juniper) 118
27-Cedarwood (Virginia) 119
28-Celery 120
29-Chamomile (German) 121
30-Chamomile (Moroccan) 122
31-Chamomile (Roman) 123
32-Cinnamon 124
33-Citronella 125
34-Coriander 126
35-Clove 127
36-Costus 128
37-Cubeb 129
38-Cumin 130
39-Cypress 131
40-Dill 132
41-Elemi 132
42-Eucalyptus 133
43-Eucalyptus (Blue Gum) 134
44-Eucalyptus (Lemon-Scented) 135
45-Fennel (Sweet) 136
46-Fir Needle 137

47-Frankincense ... 138
48-Galangal ... 139
49-Galbanum ... 140
50-Gardenia ... 141
51-Garlic ... 141
52-Geranium ... 142
53-Ginger ... 143
54-Grapefruit ... 144
55-Guaiac Wood ... 145
56-Helichrysum (Everlasting | Immortelle) ... 146
57-Hops ... 147
58-Hyacinth ... 148
59-Hyssop ... 148
60-Jasmine ... 149
61-Juniper Berry ... 150
62-Labdanum ... 151
63-Lavandin ... 152
64-Lavender ... 153
65-Lemon ... 155
66-Lemongrass ... 156
67-Lime ... 157
68-Linaloe ... 158
69-Lovage ... 159
70-Mandarin (Tangerine) ... 160
71-Marigold ... 160
72-Marjoram ... 161
73-Mastic ... 162
74-Melissa (Lemon Balm) ... 163
75-Mimosa ... 164
76-Mint (Peppermint) ... 165
77-Mint (Spearmint) ... 166
78-Myrrh ... 167
79-Narcissus ... 169
80-Neroli (Bitter Orange Blossom) ... 169
81-Niaouli ... 171
82-Nutmeg ... 172
83-Oakmoss ... 173
84-Opopanax (Hercules-All-Heal) ... 174
85-Orange (Bitter) ... 175
86-Orange (Sweet) ... 176

87-Palmarosa...... 176
88-Parsley...... 177
89-Patchouli...... 178
90-Pepper (Black)...... 179
91-Petitgrain...... 180
92-Pine (Scotch Pine)...... 181
93-Rose (Cabbage)...... 183
94-Rose (Damask)...... 184
95-Rosemary...... 185
96-Rosewood (Brazilian Rosewood)...... 187
97-Sage (Clary)...... 188
98-Sage (Spanish)...... 189
99-Sandalwood...... 190
100-Ylang-Ylang (Cananga)...... 191

Glossary Guide...... 194

BOOK-II...... 199
Recommended Remedy Recipes...... 199
Chapter 4 - Attars for Ailments...... 199

Advised Applications...... 206

Chapter 5 - Wellness & Welfare...... 208

Anxiety Alleviation & Nixing Nervousness...... 208
Creativity & Concentration...... 208
Stress Supervision...... 209
Fighting Fatigue & Leaving Lethargy...... 210
Mental & Mood Melioration...... 210
Motion Malady...... 211
Insomnia Issues & Slumber Stumpers...... 211
Menstruation & Menopausal Mitigation...... 212
Depression Deferment...... 213
Physical Pains & Acute Aches...... 214
Libido Lift...... 216
Sustained Stoppage to Smoking...... 217
Child Care & Toddler Temper Tantrums Tamer...... 218
Meditation & Mindfulness...... 220

Chapter 6 - Aesthetic Applications...... 222

Body Bulges (Cellulite Clearing | Weight Worries)...... 222
Facial Fixes (Acne | Age Spots | Chapped Lips | Wrinkles)...... 225

- Hair Hygiene (Brittleness | Dandruff | Oiliness) 226
- Skin Supplements (Oiliness & Dryness) 228
- Soak, Soap & Shampoo 229
- Nail Nourishment 231

Chapter 7 - Hearth & Home 232
- Candle Creations 232
- Cleaning Concoctions 232
- Clothing Care 233
- Fragrant Fresheners 234
- Gardening Gear (Indoor | Outdoor) 236
- Rodent Repellent (Insect | Pest) 237
- Pet Preferences 239
- Stench Suppression 240

Towards Total Transformation Through Aromatherapy: 241
A Conclusion 241

Introduction

"Using fragrance is an ideal alternative approach to alter your state of mind, mood, and life for the better, forever. It creates a pleasant aroma and aura, charm and inspiration, strength and vitality, wellness and nourishment, as well as a refined character, outlook, and bearing. In the end, it only pervades and fades in holistic positivity."
—**Lorraine McCormick**

Smell is the most primordial sense we as humans possess. The history of humanity is a living witness to the vital role our olfactory senses have served in the survival and evolution of our species.

Smelling helps us to look for our food and determine its edibility and quality. It guides us in detecting dangers, as well as discerning the safer routes. It even contributes to searching for our soulmate and identifying our loved ones.

In other words, our nose provides more for ourselves than we will ever consciously know. It may be easy to trivialize its significance in our daily lives, since much of the information for our odor-processing faculty lies in the subconscious mind.

Aromas have multifarious pieces of information processed by our brain and decoded to elicit the most appropriate response. Furthermore, our brain conveys the processed olfactory data throughout our nervous system; thereby triggering our body into fluid motion, creating and performing the various physiological responses required in any given situation.

More significantly, the crucial dimension in processing the depths of information infused by aromas in our system is the stimulation of their latent healing powers.

Aromas are derivatives of **chi**—the circulating life energy inherent in every matter. Following the ancient traditions and philosophies of Oriental medicine, the unimpeded circulation of *chi* for maintaining and sustaining the balance of positive and negative forces in our body is essential for good health; ergo, for everyone's welfare!

This is fundamentally *how* aromatherapy works it's magical healing with the use of natural essential oils. For all we know, essential oils, just like human beings, are teeming with a vital force, *chi*.

Since time immemorial, ancient and modern civilizations have been utterly delighted using a perceived elixir of life- made of aromatic botanical essential oils- and for good reason!

Essential oils possess holistic natural healing powers that enhance the physical, mental, emotional, and spiritual wellbeing while keeping everything in check through a harmonious balance.

However, it is only in recent years that the skeptic worlds of science and medicine have begun to discover, accept, and further explore how pure botanical extracts and their priceless organic chemical compounds work, potently and effectively, to influence the body, mind, and spirit for the better.

This guidebook gives due compliments to both scientific and medical communities for their recognition and acknowledgments, albeit late, on the use of essential oils for aromatherapy.

Yet, more importantly, this book shares the social responsibility to complement their research and reviews with a comprehensive reference guide and structured information towards a better learning and understanding of aromatherapy and essential oils.

"The Complete Aromatherapy Guidebook: *A Comprehensive Reference of the Natural Holistic Healing Powers of Essential Oils for Your Mind, Body, Spirit...and Comfort Zones"*—presents to you the ideal choice for what truly defines living a happy, natural, healthy, and homeopathic way of life.

This informative guidebook strategically divides its scope and intent into two extensive volumes to facilitate your learning. Within these pages, you will find a wealth of information about 100 of the best aromatherapy oils, together with 101 techniques for using them with care and confidence.

The first volume instills in you the solid foundation of a comprehensive knowledge about practicing the science and art of aromatherapy and essential oils. The second volume unveils the breadths and depths of the myriad of applications in the holistic healing spectrum of aromatherapy.

Bear in mind that with only a few drops of a dose, the potency is exceptionally grandiose! The healing holism encompasses everything about YOU—from head to toes!

© COPYRIGHT 2018 BY LORRAINE MCCORMICK
ALL RIGHTS RESERVED

In accordance with the U.S. Copyright Act of 1976, the reproduction, scanning, photocopying, recording, storing in retrieval systems, copying, transmitting, or circulating in any form by any means— electronic, mechanical, or otherwise— any part of this publication without a written permission from the publisher, constitutes piracy or theft of the author's intellectual property rights.

Exceptions only include cases of brief quotations embodied in critical reviews and/or other certain non-commercial uses permitted by copyright law. Alternatively, when using any material from this book other than reviewing simply, obtain prior permission by contacting the author, **Lorraine McCormick**.

Thank you for supporting the rights of the author and publisher.

NOTARIAL NOTES

The contents presented herein constitute the rights of the First Amendment. All information states to be truthful, accurate, reliable, and consistent. Any liability, by way of inattention or otherwise, to any use or abuse of any policies, processes, or directions contained within, is the sole discretion and responsibility of the recipient reader.

The presentation of the entire information is without a contract or any form of guarantees or assurances. Both author and publisher shall be, in no case, held liable for any fraud or fraudulent misrepresentations, monetary losses, damages, and liabilities—indirect or consequential—arising from event/s beyond reasonable control or relatively set out in this book.

Therefore, any information hereupon solely offers for educational purposes only, and as such, universal. It does not intend to be a diagnosis, prescription, or treatment for any diseases.

The Food and Drug Administration has not evaluated the statements in the book. If advice is necessary, consult a qualified professional for further questions concerning specific or critical matters on the subject.

The trademarks used herein are without any consent. Thus, the publication of the trademark is without any permission or backing by the trademark owner/s.
All trademarks/brands mentioned are for clarification purposes only and owned by the owners themselves not affiliated with the author or publisher.

BOOK—I
Essentials Of Essential Oils

Chapter 1 - Aromatherapy: An Abstract

Taking long deep breaths of your freshly ground brew of organic coffee can be a special kind of aromatherapy. Perhaps, the same goes when sticking your nose on a rose.

The scent of each natural aroma will always seem like nirvana, but what if this could be your daily mana?

You try to sniff for more, and you only recall happy memories of yore! You opt to cease smelling, and you seem to feel unwell!

Such is the wafting naked thoughts of nescience emanating from the raw perspectives of the olfactory senses.

Nonetheless, from your olfactory sense to the realms of personal beauty, nourishment, and body wellness, aromatherapy bears significantly specific definitions and purposes.

From one's crude syllogism, aromatherapy aims for healing and holism.

Aromatherapy is an essential component in every theme promoting the human mind, body, spirit, and element!

Detailed Definitions

Aromatherapy is the science and art of applying herbal essential oils to stimulate, relax, and keep your mind, body, and spirit in a harmonious balance. These ***essential oils*** are pure, natural concentrates extracted from the entirety of a plant, or the specific sections that contain the most aromatic and potent properties.

The extraction process produces the host plant's essential oil concentrate, which is typically 75% to 100% more concentrated than the dried herb. The neat concentrate contains rich organic compounds with a much-concentrated vigor.

This inherent vital energy of essential oils provides the potent natural healing powers found in aromatherapy. They facilitate and augment sustained maintenance of your intended enhancements—whether for beauty and physicality, mood and emotion, lifestyle, cognition, general health, wellbeing, or every nook and cranny of your comfort zones.

Nevertheless, an essential oil is exceptionally more than merely a highly concentrated botanical extract. It is neither fatty nor greasy, as you might have initially perceived it to be.

Much less, it does not refer to a certain *need*. Rather, it denotes the *real essence* of a plant's intrinsic scent. In a more definitive perspective, an essential oil is characteristically the blood, the life force, and the soul of its mother plant. In which case, it is the holy ghost of the whole host plant!

The key attribute of an essential oil is its distinctive fragrance. Equally important is that it loads itself with the originated plant's medicinal, therapeutic, cosmetic qualities, as well as other beneficial characteristics.

Sometimes referred to as *volatile oils,* essential oils are sensitive to light and heat. They are also renowned as *ethereal oils* because of their delicateness, lightness, which is attributed to microscopic molecular structures stored in cellular vessels within the plant. For these reasons, they are easily prone to evaporation.

Like fine wines, essential oils can vary from season to season due to environmental factors like weather. Farming and cultivation procedures of the host plants can also be critically accountable for causing the degeneration of the properties of essential oils, and for good reason! As the old cliché goes, *"a rotten tree bears bad fruit."*

Applying essential oils as a form of natural healing is both gentle and effective. They can easily absorb into your system by applying them in a multitude of ways. Oftentimes, it is the first line of defense a natural medicine health practitioner or herbalist will rely on and use prior to subsequently performing more invasive treatments.

On one hand, most professional practitioners apply approximately 300 essential oils for treating a broad range of bodily ailments. On the other hand, many long-time home practitioners would generally use around 10 to 20 essential oils on a regular schedule.

Among the most popular and commonly used natural essential oils are chamomile, clary sage, eucalyptus, lavender, and orange. Of course, you can also use them on yourself, your family and friends, or even in the comforts of your room and home- indeed, you will witness a great difference!

Recorded Roots & Anecdotal Accounts

The therapeutic application of aromatic plants and herbs, as well as their respective essential oils, dates back to the dawn of time. The earliest evidence of these botanical therapeutic practices were the discovery of several wall paintings and hieroglyphics inside the fabled caves of Lascaux in France, carbon-dated to about 18,000 B.C.

These archaeological findings only proved to indicate that prehistoric humans already had an understanding of the natural healing powers of plants. Clearly, they had been using botanical medicines on a daily basis for several hundreds of centuries.

Although the first distillation process of essential oils was quite vague, it is apparent that many ancient cultures and civilizations have their own accounts of these wonder-oils of nature. Records affirmed that ancient Egyptians were among the first to use pure and high-quality essential oils in 4,500 B.C.

They considered these herbal extracts, sometimes traded with pure gold, as sacred. Only members of royalty and high priests had the exclusive authority of using them.

In fact, each of the Egyptian deities has an assigned signature blend of essential oils. They used an assortment of unique essential oil concoctions during religious ceremonies, intimacies, meditations, and even during preparations for war.

Sometime in 3,000 B.C., Hindu gurus in India developed a health science and medicine called *Ayurveda*. This ancient medical discipline anchored deeply on maintaining balance among the five essential elements: earth, water, air, fire, and ether.

The elemental ether covered the natural remedial potions that contained a vast collection of pure essential oils. As a testimonial, the Vedic literature listed more than 700 curative botanical agents used in *Ayurvedic* healing.

In China, the legendary deity, Huang Di, also known as the Yellow Emperor (2698–2598 B.C.), constructed a comprehensive medical reference book, '*Suwen*.' with the help of his ministers. The esoteric scripture became the encompassing foundation for both actual and theoretical principles of the highly revered Traditional Chinese Medicine (TCM).

Suwen notated, in broad details, hundreds of essential oils and aromatic herbs as immediate remedies for a host of ailments. The medical text remained significantly relevant up into present times, since most Oriental medicine practitioners continue to refer to and base their alternative medicine treatment practices on this book, especially on the myriad of health benefits attributed to aromatic essential oils.

In addition to its universal recognition, the Christian Bible has cited for more than 200 references to the use of essential oils. The Holy Scripture mentioned them primarily for their religious purposes, the sheer delight of their fragrances, and their values as royal presents- as manifested by the wise men's gifts of myrrh and frankincense to the newborn Messiah.

Roman and Greek ancients also show early documentation of the use of essential oils. In most cases, they apply these botanical oils for aromatic therapy, personal care and hygiene, medicine, and therapeutic massage or reflexology.

Circa 500 to 400 B.C. saw the creation of volumes of literature furnished by *'The Father of Medicine,'* Hippocrates. These documents featured more than 300 plant species and their essential oils, as well as their respective medicinal effects. In one passage, Hippocrates lectures that a daily perfumed bath, coupled by a scented massage, is the enlightened way towards good health.

Another influential Greek physician, Galen, manifested his extensive knowledge of the medical aspects of essential oils. He composed the voluminous

'Galenic Medicine,' which included several plant species categorized into various medicinal applications.

The treasured books of Hippocrates and Galen ultimately found their way into Persia after Rome fell. They saw themselves translated into several languages and became the primary reference, and fundamental principle, of both the Pakistani and Iranian, or Islamic, Traditional Medicines (ITM).

The Iranian polymath, Abu Ali Ibn Sina, popularly known as Avicenna, cataloged an estimated 800 botanical species. He described in painstaking detail each of their effects on the human body. The field of aromatherapy credited him for refining and recording the first traditional extraction procedures of pure and high-grade essential oils from aromatic botanicals.

The Western world only accessed firsthand knowledge of herbal medicine and essential oils after European Crusade knights journeyed into the Middle East. As result, several Crusade armies started carrying herbal extracts and wearing perfumes. Others obtained the technical skills and know-how of extracting the aromatic oils.

During the bubonic plague in the Late Middle Ages (1340–1400), Europe's desperate doctors adopted *Ayurvedic* treatments from the East with success. They specifically used efficacious essential oil blends as primary alternatives to their ineffective medicines.

In the 16th century, medieval alchemists who sought the *quintessence*—the panacea and secret of life—have found many plant's aromatic oil as a vital elixir. They were the first to conceive the term, **"essential oil"** and regarded them as the *fifth element,* after earth, wind, water, and fire (as in the *Ayurvedic* way).

These elements related to nature, as well as the consciousness and physical beings of humans. Medieval alchemists believed that essential oils complemented the formation of the heavenly body—our true life force!

In 1653, the English botanist, Nichols Culpeper, presented detailed treatments for numerous medical conditions throughout his book, *"Complete Herbal."* It contained a trove of herbal and pharmaceutical knowledge on preparing and dispensing venerable tonics, which contained essential oils blended with other efficient plant-based compounds, which are predominant applications to this day.

At the early turn of the 20th century, the French chemist, Rene-Maurice Gattefosse, discovered the swift and potent natural healing qualities of essential oils after he burnt his hand in a laboratory accident and treated the injury with lavender's essential oil. Eventually, he coined the modern-day era term, ***"aromatherapy"*** after performing further research on the therapeutic qualities of lavender's essential oil and before offering it to the various medical institutions in France.

During World War II, the French practitioner of aromatherapy, Dr. Jean-Valnet, used essential oils of therapeutic grades for the treatment of the injured soldiers. A couple of Valnet's students, Dr. Jean-Claude Lapraz and Dr. Paul Belaiche, probed for more proof on the successful treatments.

They conducted extensive research and qualitative analyses about the analgesic, antibacterial, antifungal, anti-inflammatory, antispasmodic, antiseptic, and antiviral properties of essential oils. Eureka! Truly, both concluded in unison that these powerful natural substances bear substantial healing abilities.

Concept and Context

Essential oils are very much different from other common pharmaceutical chemicals and substances used for healing and nourishment. Since their molecules—containing highly active organic compounds—are microscopic, they can easily permeate through dermal layers.

More interestingly, due to their infinitesimal size and dimension, they can even infiltrate through the seemingly impervious *blood-brain barrier* mechanism. This denotes the filtering dynamics of blood capillaries, which supply blood to your brain and spinal cord tissues and block the passage of certain infiltrating substances.

Therefore, you can easily reap their positive effects and benefits by simply administering a topical application. Incidentally, these molecules are the principal reason for essential oils having their own unique fragrances and their amazing ability to scent an entire room so pleasantly, even with only a single minuscule drop!

Appropriate Administration

Performing aromatherapy and its techniques involve a variety of tactical procedures. Yet, with countless available essential oils, it can truly be confusing for any beginner on how to administer each of the essential oils in fitting manners; or, in the most suitable, convenient, and comfortable ways.

For proper guidance, you will only have THREE fundamental methods for the appropriate administration of essential oils in aromatherapy:

● **External** – covers the different types of topical administration—massage or friction, neat-on acupuncture or reflexology points, and compress—for applying the various herbal essential oil products in the form of bath soaps, creams, lotions, lip balms, salves, salts, insect repellants, tinctures, etc.

⚫ **Inhalation** – involves the application of steam inhalation, nasal sprays, perfumes, candles, room sprays, potpourri burners, and diffusers

⚫ **Internal** – prescribes the ingestion of capsules, charcoal or lactose tablets, vegetable oils, apple cider vinegar, honey, food suppositories, and herbal teas and brews

Regardless of what specific applications you use, the essential oil's molecules, which contain a sea of potent chemical compounds, will guarantee a complete penetration and absorption into your entire body. As they plunge into and journey along your bloodstream, they begin to perform like an orchestra, interacting in perfect harmony with various body cells, tissues, and organs.

The molecules bind compatibly with your skin and nail tissues, blood and blood vessels, joints, muscles and their connective tissues, sensory nerves, sweat and sebaceous glands, and hair follicles. These organic interactions are impossible to duplicate or reproduce, even synthetically. For, after all, they are the magical workings of the wonders of nature!

In effect, the molecules promptly stimulate a range of physical, psychological, physiological, and emotional responses. Essentially, the efficacious results run the gamut of a natural holistic healing!

CONSTITUENT COMPOSITION

Essential oils compose powerful principal, auxiliary, and trace components classified into three major categories—*monoterpenes, sesquiterpenes,* and *phenylpropanes*—with each category classified further into sub-categorical molecular compounds (refer to Image-1):

MONOTERPENES		
MOLECULE TYPE	EFFECTS	CHIEF EXAMPLES
Monoterpenes Hydrocarbons	Stimulant	Orange, Pine
Ketones	Mucolytic	Rosemary, Sage
Aldehydes	Calmative	Melissa, Citronella
Esters	Antispasmodic	Clary Sage, Lavender
Alcohols	Natural Tonic	Peppermint, Palmarosa
Phenols	Irritant, Stimulant	Oregano, Thyme
SESQUITERPENES		
Sesquiterpenes Hydrocarbons	Anti-inflammatory	German Chamomile
Alcohols	Various	Sandalwood, Vetiver
Lactones	Mucolytic	Laurel
PHENYLPROPANES		
Estragol	Antispasmodic	Tarragon
Anethol	Antispasmodic	Anise
Eugenol	Sensitizing	Clove
Cinnamic Aldehyde	Antiseptic	Cinnamon, Cassia

Image-1: Categorical Components of Essential Oils

These specific chemical components and their primary effects will ultimately form your fundamental scientific knowledge and understanding of essential oils. Moreover, they will be your main reference for the appropriate applications of the essential oils amidst your engagements with the art of aromatherapy.

Nevertheless, as soon as you have a good grasp and the hang of these constituent compositions of essential oil molecules, they will inevitably lead you to the most exciting world of the aromatherapy program. Exciting as it can be, you will eventually have your shining moment to formulate your own signature essential oil recipe, prepared and concocted as your personalized healing lotion, salve, scent, soap, spray, tincture, perfume, candle, etc.

Product Potencies

Because essential oils are richly concentrated, a small vial, or even a single drop, will certainly go a very long way. It's like tossing a tiny pebble in a calm pond- you will subsequently see how the entire surface of water reacts with a rippling effect.

For using much less, the coverage seems boundless. That is how efficiently and effectively potent an essential oil is!

For instance, just a single drop of peppermint essential oil equates to about 28 to 30 cups of peppermint tea! Dispensing such minute quantities applies across the administrative and functional versatilities of essential oils (refer to Image-2 for further examples).

Administration	Potency Amount	Ideal Essential Oil
Bath, Compress, Body Wash	Add **6-8 drops** to a basin or tub filled with warm water	Ylang-Ylang, Peppermint, Geranium, Orange, Roman Chamomile, Frankincense
Spa Facial Steam	Add **8-12 drops** to a pan of heated water; tent your head over with a towel	Chamomile, Fennel, Eucalyptus, Geranium, Lavender, Parsley
Reflexology, Friction, Massage	Add **6-8 drops** to 1-oz. of carrier oil or a derivative organic plant oil	Thyme, Lemongrass, Peppermint, Rosemary, Lavender
Basic Inhalation	Add **2-5 drops** to a cotton ball or tissue paper (store in a sealed case after using)	Eucalyptus, Peppermint, Tea Tree, Lavender
Smelling Salts	Add **10 drops** to 1-tsp of rock salt (store in a sealed case after using)	Basil, Peppermint, Rosemary (or a mixed combo of them)
Chest Decongestant	Add **1-13 drops** per 2-cups of heated water in a basin and inhale the vapor	Eucalyptus, Peppermint, Frankincense, Oregano, Cinnamon, Geranium
Liquid Mist, Spray	Add **3-5 drops** to 1-tsp of alcohol and purified water in an atomizer	Peppermint, Lavender, Witch Hazel
Diffusion	Apply **1-2 drops** on a cool light bulb or in a ceramic diffuser	Peppermint, Eucalyptus, Marjoram, Lavender, Neroli, Citrus, Chamomile, Juniper
Perfume	Add **25 drops** to 1-oz. of perfumed or denatured alcohol (shake before use)	Any of your favorite combination

Image-2: Sample Coverages of A Few Possible Essential Oil Applications

Bonuses & Benefits

As its terminology simply implies, aromatherapy is the healing power of scents. Many aromatic essential oils provide and complement the therapeutic dimension of aromatherapy.

With almost a thousand identified aromatic essential oils, a list of each of their delightful and therapeutic benefits can be never-ending! Nonetheless, the bottom line is that essential oils result in a powerful natural healing, whether administered internally, externally or by inhalation.

Aromatherapy—through using essential oils—is a type of holistic healing. It embraces to wholly benefit wide scopes and interdependent aspects of your personal beauty, hygiene, body nourishment, wellness, and total health care.

The beneficial holism of aromatherapy extends to your daily home living, individuality, lifestyle, and even to your pockets (or wherewithal), so to speak. The following is a bird's eye view of a dozen well-loved, well-researched, and scientifically supported bonuses and benefits you gain for practicing aromatherapy with essential oils:

♦ **Help Harnessing Hormones:** Hormones are useful organic chemical compounds produced by the *endocrine glands* (i.e., ovary, adrenal gland, testes, pancreas, pineal gland, thyroid, and pituitary glands). Essential oils collaborate harmoniously with your glands by helping to efficiently release hormones into your bloodstream.

In turn, blood vessels convey these freshly released hormones to various cells, tissues, and organs throughout your body. Hormones will then stimulate and positively influence the physiological activities of your body, and thereby trigger a normal and balanced regulation of your metabolism, progressive tissue growths, cell regeneration, and other bodily functions.

For many essential oils, they direct their energies into controlling your hormones to their optimum levels. Primarily, they enable the reduction of cortisol hormone levels, which result in mood enhancements and reduced depression symptoms.

They also tend to heighten your testosterone hormone level, which incline engendering love and intensifying sexual desires. For this reason, many consider essential oils to be a reliable aphrodisiac.

A 2017 publication in the *"Neuro Endocrinology Journal"* indicated that several essential oils, notably **rose** and **geranium**, influence estrogen hormone concentrations in women's saliva. This proved to be beneficial for women experiencing menopausal symptoms, which are typical consequences of diminished levels of estrogen hormone secretion.

Geranium and **clary sage** oils are effective in improving conditions such as *polycystic ovary syndrome* (PCOS) and infertility, including *premenstrual syndrome* (PMS) and menstruation symptoms.

♦ **Improve Immunity & Inhibit Inflammatory Infections:** In light of growing threat of antibiotic resistance in the field of modern healthcare, several essential oils can serve as either a singular or combination therapy to combat bacterial infections and anti-inflammatory symptoms in a safer and more natural way.

These essential oils possess antibacterial, anti-fungal, anti-inflammatory, antiseptic, and antiviral properties. The common organic chemical substances in these essential oils, like *terpenes*, *esters*, *phenols*, and *ketones*, have the potential to destroy foreign and harmful *pathogens* (i.e., fungi, virus, and bacteria) that threaten your health.

Some ideal essential oils for improving your immunity are **cinnamon**, **eucalyptus**, **frankincense**, **ginger**, **lemon**, **myrrh**, **oregano**, and **peppermint**.

♦ **Develop Desirable Digestions:** Essential oils for digestion augment the functions of the digestive system. Foremost, they facilitate the digestion process by stimulating enzymes that are responsible for breaking down and absorbing ingested *macronutrients* (i.e., carbohydrates, fats, proteins).

At the same time, these typical essential oils promote the elimination of waste matter. They also help to relieve gastrointestinal related issues such as abdominal pains or stomach-aches, constipation, stomach gas spasms, upset stomach, nausea, ulcers, and even *internal bowel syndrome* (IBS).

The *"World Journal of Gastroenterology"* published a study confirming the use of **ginger** oil as an effective reliever to most of the aforementioned gastrointestinal conditions. Additionally, the study recommended **peppermint** oil to provide a swift relief from IBS symptoms.

Other helpful essential oils for developing desirable digestions are **black pepper**, **fennel**, **marjoram**, **lemongrass**, and **juniper**.

♦ **Enhance Energy Extents:** Not only do certain essential oils bolster your energy levels, but they also improve athletic abilities and physical performances. Some oils have stimulating effects to increase the oxygen supply to the brain, and thereby allowing you to be more creative, focused, cognizant, and alert while allowing a more refreshed, revitalized, and energized feeling.

The *"Journal of the International Society of Sports Nutrition"* recently published results of studies conducted on **peppermint** oil relative to athletic performances. The study confirmed that the essential oil has a potent ability to increase concentrations of oxygen in the brain.

Using peppermint oil can also improve physical exercise performances as well as reducing feelings of exhaustion and lethargy, especially in healthy male athletes who take peppermint oil diluted with water for 10 straight days.

Alternative essential oils for boosting energy include ***lemon***, ***eucalyptus***, ***grapefruit***, ***lemongrass***, and ***rosemary***.

⬥ **Suppress Stresses & Abort Anxieties:** Among the most renowned benefits of most essential oils is the ability to uplift moods, truly altering negative emotions for the better.

On one hand, some essential oils suppress stress and depression, rather they induce feelings of peacefulness, relaxation, and calmness. On the other hand, they dispel anger and quell anxieties, as well as helping to build confidence and stimulate motivations.

A 2014 study assessed the effectiveness of aromatherapy for 82 elderly patients diagnosed with depression, anxiety, and chronic pain symptoms. Researchers found that after a month's treatment, all of the patients experienced drastic reductions in their negative emotions.

In another recent study entitled, *"Complementary Therapies in Clinical Practice,"* aromatherapy has been shown as a complemental therapy for reducing depression and anxiety levels, especially in women after giving birth.

This study further suggested that the best essential oils to relieve stress, depression, and anxiety are ***ylang-ylang, bergamot, Roman chamomile, vetiver, lavender, orange***, and ***frankincense***.

- **Boost Brainpower Behaviors:** The calming, sedative and neuroprotective effects of some essential oils are among the most impressive benefits. These effects help to accelerate the learning processes, boost memory, and maintain focus and attention for longer periods of time.

Generally, they improve the overall cognitive performances. Besides, they have been helpful to many patients afflicted by various neurodegenerative disorders such as dementia and Alzheimer's disease- including the agitation fits arising from these conditions.

To support such claims, the paper *"Frontiers in Aging Neuroscience"* published a scientific review emphasizing the composition and functions of powerful antioxidants in essential oils. Researchers noted that these special components work to inhibit the scavenging tendencies of free radicals in the brain.

In other words, they help prevent outsets of inflammatory brain diseases. As a result, they naturally improve the brain's faculties and functions.

Both sedative and stimulating essential oils can be useful for boosting brainpower behaviors. **Lavender** and **peppermint** are the leading therapeutic oils for realizing this benefit.

◆ **<u>Palliate Pains & Alleviate Aches:</u>** Researchers reviewed a dozen studies on using specific essential oils that bear pain relief benefits. In the end, all turned out positive results.

Of these studies, a publication in *"Pain Research and Treatment"* summarized that aromatherapy has more significant effects than those of placebo-controlled treatments applied for pain reduction and relief. The selected essential oils were even helpful in treating gynecological, obstetrical, and post-operative pains.

They were also beneficial for soothing an assortment of common body pains suffered by the elderly, such as nerve pains, muscle cramps, and lower back pains. Moreover, rigid aromatherapy programs were able to relieve rheumatoid arthritis and inflammatory symptoms felt in various joints of the body such as the fingers, toes, neck, knees, spine, and hips.

Fact is that several essential oils possess superior analgesic qualities such as **chamomile**, **ginger**, **eucalyptus**, **frankincense**, **lavender**, **myrrh**, **marjoram**, **peppermint**, **rosemary**, and **turmeric**.

♦ **<u>Support Skincare & Hair Health:</u>** One of the safest, most natural, and effective ways to maintain your personal beauty and body care regimens is using essential oils for aromatherapy. Many essential oils improve the overall appearances of your skin, nails, and hair by acting simultaneously as an astringent, moisturizer, and toner.

They can also slow acne growths, abate the early signs of aging such as age spots and wrinkles, relieve irritated skin, and shield your skin from harmful ultraviolet rays. In addition, these beauty care essential oils can also aid to inhibit inflammatory skin conditions such as lupus, eczema, and dermatitis. They can even heal wounds such as minor cuts, slits, swellings, bruises, and abrasions.

All of these skin benefits stem from the ability of essential oils to fight pathogens responsible for various dermatological infections. Several reviews, which attested these effects, also found essential oils to be beneficial for hair growth.

A 2015 study approved the efficacy of ***rosemary*** oil on patients suffering from alopecia, or hair loss. Aside from promoting rapid hair growth, they can also be used to thicken and strengthen hair.

A published study from the *"Evidence-Based Complementary and Alternative Medicine"* further stated that it identified and recommended 90 specific essential oils with about 1,500 combinations for effective general dermatological health applications.

Among the most notable essential oils supporting skincare are ***clary sage***, ***Roman chamomile***, ***frankincense***, ***geranium***, ***myrrh***, ***helichrysum***, ***lavender***, and ***rosemary.***

♦ **Terminate Toxicity:** Nowadays, we seem to feel helpless, inhaling thousands of toxins from our polluted environment. Sometimes, we become unaware and gullible, ingesting an abundance of chemically derived substances in our foods. These are just a few typical staples of our modern ways of living.

Of course, toxins imminently pose as real dangers to our health. However, we can be safe upon dwelling in the sanctuary of aromatherapy. The versatility of some essential oils not only promotes detoxification in our body but also in our homes as well.

As discussed previously, some essential oils facilitate digestion, which promotes the natural process of detoxification. Other essential oils function as mild diuretics. Hence, they contribute to increased urine production- and thereby improve the body's natural detoxification process.

Applying detoxifying essential oils can help flush out toxins that build up in the body. In the same way of cleansing your body, they can also purify the circulating air in your home or in your workplace.

The organic disinfectant qualities of these essential oils can clean and refresh the ambiance of your comfort zones in a more natural way by destructing harmful pollutants and pathogens. Compared to most traditional home cleaning products, which contain harmful chemicals, essential oils only contain safe organic compounds.

For promoting internal detoxification, studies advise using essential oils of *fennel*, *ginger*, *grapefruit*, *lemon*, *lemongrass*, *parsley*, and *peppermint*.

Excellent essential oils suggested for terminating toxicity in your home or workplace are *cinnamon*, *eucalyptus*, *grapefruit*, *lemongrass*, *lemon*, *orange*, and *peppermint*.

⬥ **Hinder Headaches and Mitigate Migraines:** Most of the basic painkillers on the market relieve headaches and migraines by simply masking the real cause of the pain. In the case of essential oils, they work to the root and address the main cause of the problem.

Essential oils for headaches not only provide pain relief but also reduce stress and improve air or blood circulation. Stress, congested nasal airways, and constricted flows of blood are typically the major causes for developing headaches and migraines.

A 2012 clinical trial evaluated the effectiveness of inhaling lavender oil for 15 minutes during a period of 2 hours against a placebo-controlled therapy for the treatment of both headaches and migraines. The test showed statistically significant decreases in pain severities and symptomatic aches for the participants responding to the essential oil.

Apart from **lavender**, other helpful essential oils are **peppermint**, which can stimulate blood flow and produce a cooling effect; **rosemary**, which can promote balanced circulation with a calming effect while reducing inflammation; and, **eucalyptus**, which can relieve the buildup of trapped air pressures in the sinus by clearing the nasal airways.

⬥ **Reform Rest & Recreation Routines:** Sedating essential oils are helpful for people who suffer from insomnia. Specifically, **lavender** oil is the most effective in addressing sleep issues and promoting an undisturbed rest or sleep. This is because lavender has the ability to help you feel calm and relaxed.

Numerous studies, testimonials, and pieces of evidence have point to the relaxant property of lavender oil. It owns a popular repute to be an inexpensive, non-invasive, and easily applicable intervention for people who have trouble sleeping or experience anxieties.

With a corrected sleeping habits, former insomniacs can rearrange and manage their daily schedules and become more productive. As a result, they could also enjoy spending quality time both resting and enjoying recreational activities.

Lavender oil, though, is not alone in reforming routines towards productivity. **Bergamot**, **ylang-ylang**, **Roman chamomile**, and **vetiver** oils are also effective alternatives to lavender oil's abilities.

♦ **Enduring Economics:** In summary, aside from using essential oils for aromatherapy to prevent and heal ailments, they are far less expensive than any modern medical treatments, or other preferred ways and means of achieving the similar effective benefits aforementioned. With essential oils, you can easily maintain and sustain their applications over the long haul without ever hurting your wallet.

Essential oils have the added bonus of being pure, organic, and all natural! Those familiar pricey products you have been using all this time often contains impurities and chemical or synthetic substances that may be harmful to your body.

If products compromised you with their health hazards, it would be the height of misfortune. You do not only feel sore and sorry for dispensing steeper costs for them, but you will certainly feel sorer and sorrier dispensing other steeper costs at a dispensary!

As mentioned, a single drop of an essential oil stretches its effective services and mileage to some lengthy extents. If you compare its more economical coverage against the rest of its counterparts, then you will definitely subscribe to the essential oil's cost and cause—less is more!

Chapter 2 - Art of Aromatherapy: Abiding Advised Approaches

For any aromatherapy practitioner, whether they are would-be, beginner, aficionado, enthusiast, professional expert, or you—it is crucially necessary to know the techniques and methodologies for an appropriate administration, production, procurement, dosage, storage duration, dilution, combination, concoction, and the safest aromatherapy practices.

Else, a sniff gets you stiff! Ergo, learn each step!

Each of these are integral to embracing the science and art of aromatherapy. Abide by the following advised approaches:

Production Processes

Foremost, disabuse your mind from the common misconception of producing an essential oil. You do not actually *make* an essential oil; but rather, you must *extract* it!

Extraction aims to obtain a certain plant's most active and potent elemental compounds, which function as the plant's élan vital, meaning spirit or vital force. In essence, it is the liquefied version of the source plant.

The vital force of a source plant can find refuge on its flower, fruit, leaf, seed, root, bark, twig, rind, and resin. You can only draw it out through its specifically required extraction method.

The principal methods of extracting essential oils include steam distillation, water distillation, water-steam distillation, cold-press extraction, and solvent extraction. Solvent extraction covers the processes of carbon dioxide extraction, maceration, and the cold and hot enfleurage.

⦁ **Steam-Distillation:** Isolating the essential oil from its source plant through steam-distillation is the most commonly applied extraction method. Its popularity hinges on the principle that it effectively allows for a separation process at lower temperatures through the introduction of steam.

Heating to the boiling points is never an option so the process does not decompose the essential oil; but rather, it protects and preserves the integrity of the highly volatile and heat-sensitive organic compounds such as aromatic botanicals (refer to Image-3).

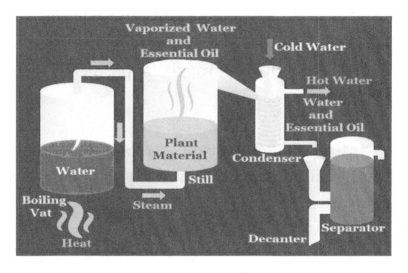

Image-3: Schematic Diagram of a Steam-Distillation Extraction Process

◆ **Water-Distillation:** Some plant materials, specifically the flower petals of orange blossoms and roses, are extremely fragile and delicate. When introducing steam into the distillation processes, they have the tendency of clumping together, and thus, hindering the extraction of optimum yields.

Hence, the most effective extraction method, in this case, is doing away with the still, and instead submerging the plant materials in purified water inside the boiling vat. The vaporized water and essential oil go directly to the condenser, where the condensed emulsion cools down and pours into the separator (refer back to Image-3).

Purified water protects the extracted essential oil from overheating and the boiling process prevents the plant materials from clumping. The water remaining in the vat is usually fragrant; and as such, reusable. Often referred to by many terms such as *hydrosol, herbal water, herbal distillate, floral water,* or *essential water,* it is a common ingredient in room sprays and skincare products.

- **Water-Steam Distillation:** This extraction method combines both water- and steam-distillation processes, where it immerses the plant material in purified water inside the still. The boiling vat feeds steam to the still.

- **Cold Press Extraction:** Also termed as *scarification* or *expression*, the cold press extraction method is the original process for extracting essential oils, prior to the discovery of distillation. The process usually derives essential oils from the fresh rinds or peelings of citrus fruits.

The process begins by placing whole fruits (of the desired essential oil) in a mechanical device, which pierces them to rupture the fruit's oil sacs located on the rind's underside. The piercing or scarification process prepares the fruit for pressing to squeeze out its essential oils and juices.

The produced liquid emulsion, which still contains solid particles like crushed pulps and peels, undergo a filtration process through centrifugation. Not only does centrifugation separate the solids from liquids but it also separates the juice layer from the essential oil. The extraction process ends with siphoning off or decanting the essential oil into another receptacle.

♦ **<u>Solvent Extraction:</u>** Interchangeably termed as *'liquid extraction'*, this method uses food-grade solvents such as ethanol and hexane to isolate essential oils from plant material. The extraction process produces a finer fragrance compared to any type of distillation processes.

This extraction method is ideally suitable for plant materials that are mainly resinous (i.e., the bark of the frankincense tree); extremely delicate aromatics with lower resistance to distress and pressure of steam distillation, and typically yielding lesser quantities of essential oils.

Treating a solvent to the plant material produces *'concrete'*—a waxy aromatic substance that releases essential oils when blended with alcohol and introduced to heat, technically termed as *'vacuum distillation.'* However, traces of the solvent remain in the essential oil, used commonly in perfumery.

- **Carbon Dioxide (CO_2) Extraction:** This extraction process introduces CO_2 gas in its *'supercritical state,'* which is subjecting the gas to a pressure higher than its critical values. The pressurized CO_2 gains liquid-like properties as well as gaseous, and is pumped into an extraction chamber.

Due to the liquid and gaseous properties CO_2, it acts as a solvent on the plant matter, extracting the essential oils as well as other substances. The essential oil content simply dissolves into the liquid CO_2.

The complete separation of CO_2 from the extracted oil is done by activating the pressure release valve of the extraction chamber. CO2 goes back to its normal pressure and evaporates, returning to its gaseous state (refer to Image-4).

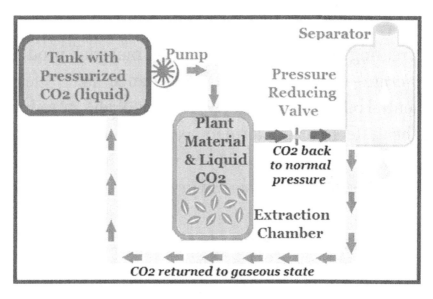

Image-4: Schematic Diagram of Carbon Dioxide Extraction Process

The CO_2 gas solvent is odorless and colorless. It is what humans exhale and what plants require for their sustenance and survival.

This only denotes the harmlessness of the CO_2 solvent in the extraction process. CO_2 operates under temperatures of 95°F-100°F (35°C-38°) unlike the higher temperatures of 140°F to 212°F (60 to 100) applied in steam-distillation.

Essential oils obtained through steam-distillation have varying qualities. These qualitative changes are dependent on the pressures, temperatures, and duration applied during the process.

In contrast, essential oils derived from the CO_2 extraction method possess higher qualities since the process does not apply heat. Heat alters the molecular composition as well as certain qualities of the plant material and extracted oil.

Therefore, the qualities of the resulting essential oil from the CO_2 extraction process remain *'denatured'* (no alterations from its natural state) and resemble more the composite qualities of the original plant material. For further comparisons, CO_2 extracts are more viscous, thick, and fragrant than distilled essential oils.

- **Maceration:** Macerated essential oils, also referred to as *infused oils*, are extractions from the therapeutic properties of a plant material. The maceration method introduces a solvent, *menstruum* (a commonly used solvent in the preparation of a drug) for the extraction process.

Menstruum has the efficiency to extract larger and heavier plant molecules. In other words, the extracted oil captures more essences and beneficial properties of the host plant. This is the chief advantage of macerated oils over distilled oils.

The maceration process starts by drying the ideal plant material for infusion. Drying must ensure zero moisture content- otherwise, any traces of moisture will encourage microbial growths or cause rancidity to the oil.

Macerated essential oils become cloudy and stinky when rancid. However, adding 5% vitamin E-rich wheat germ oil or vitamin E oil can prevent rancidity.

Drying also prepares the plant material for easy cutting, crushing, or grounding, allowing plant material to be turned into a moderately coarse powder. You can perform the next step of the procedure as follows:

♦ Place the powdered material in a vessel and add the solvent. Close the vessel and allow the mixture to stand for a week, shaking it occasionally.

♦ Strain the liquid mixture. Press the *marc* (solid residue) to recover and juice out any remaining liquid.

♦ Mix the strained and expressed liquids. Clarify the liquid through filtration or *subsidence* (allowing a gradual sinking or settling down of fine particles in the mixture).

♦ Store the filtered liquid in an airtight container in a cool, dry place for up to a year.

♦ **Enfleurage (Cold & Hot):** As one of the oldest methods of extracting essential oils, enfleurage is no longer commonly in use. Nonetheless, it remains worthy to recall its significance to emphasize the role of solvents and their infusion with botanical material in extracting essential oils.

The enfleurage process had its heyday in ancient perfumery. It implements purified and odorless fats and oils derived from vegetables or animals—usually tallow or lard—to absorb the fragrance of fresh flowers.

The process starts by spreading out the fat and setting it over glass plates along a frame called a *chassis*. On top of the fat layer, fresh flower petals or whole flowers are set for 1 to 3 days, or for 2 weeks, depending on the flower species used.

During this time, their fragrance seeps into the fat. The seeping process only ends when the fat reaches the desired saturation levels of absorption.

The fragrance-saturated fat is a crude product called *enfleurage pomade*. The process continues when separating botanical extracts from the remaining fat by washing the *pomade* with alcohol.

Soap making processes reuse the remaining fat. As the alcohol evaporates from the infused mixture, the final product is the *absolute,* or the purest quality.

Performing the enfleurage method can be either a cold or cold process. The hot process follows the same procedures except fats are heated.

Blending Basics

Blending, or pairing essential oils drop by drop is an art. It is all about inhaling per se! Among the best ways to start creating your personal fragrances, especially if you are a beginner, is through trial and error-experimenting! Combine essential oils that might have struck your innermost senses, cast a spell on you, enchanted you, or caused you to fall in love at first inhalation.

Each of us is unique, and each of us connects or relates differently to certain fragrances, just as each of our memories associating with that fragrance will vary. Concocting aromatherapy blends is truly an intimate, personal, and creative activity. Therefore, it helps to recall, as always, by begin blending essential oils you love before branching out and creating blends for others.

Now, this may give rise to an obstacle and cause you to abort your launch right from the very start. ***How then do you identify aromatic notes?***

The primary skill you ought to develop is to recognize the songs of scent, know their notes! In the same language that musicians identify the tones of a melody into musical notes of chords, aromatherapists and perfumers catalog aromas of individual essential oils and blends into three fundamental components or *notes*— top, middle, and base note.

It is noteworthy to know that oils and blends can possess components of all three *notes*. Nonetheless, experts classify such oils on their most dominant note.

⬥ **Top Note** – It is the initial prominent impression of a blend. Oftentimes, it is the typical feature of the oil. It has a sharp tone, but the fragrance does not last long as it springs swiftly from the aroma.

⬥ **Middle or Body Note** – Commonly referred to as the *bouquet* or *heart* of the aroma, it characterizes the fragrance of an essential oil to last longer: for about 1-2 hours on a perfume-testing strip.

♦ **Base Note or Fixative** – This scent appears or exudes much later compared to the top and middle notes. Known also as the *dry out* note, it can appear a few hours to even an entire day after the perfume-testing strip is dry.

The base note provides the staying power to a blend. It is what powerful base notes provide to soaps to help maintain their long-lasting fragrances. Thus, the base note allows you to determine the enduring capability of your essential oil blend.

NOTE: Never confuse or misinterpret base note with base oil. The base oil is a fixed oil applied to dilute essential oils.

When blending, select aromatic oils from each category. Think of it as if creating a musical rhythm, as if composing the aroma chords for your song of scent!

As an exercise, begin choosing the essential oils you believe will produce a delightful aromatherapy blend.

Start inhaling...get creative! Worry not about which notes you choose. Keep it basic: select five essential oils as a start and perform the following exercise:

Concocting Combination Calisthenics

⬥ Aroma Acquaintanceship & Noting Notes:

⬥ **Step-1:** Think about what fragrances you naturally like. Try asking yourself whether you enjoy the zest of an herb or spice, long for the scent of a certain flower, or love the green and crisp aromas of nature. This helps you to choose the appropriate essential oils for your intended blend.

⬥ **Step-2:** Perform a sensory test, or an olfaction analysis, on your chosen oils. On a perfume-testing strip, place 1-drop from each essential oil. Draw the strip gradually to your nose, as if circumscribing imaginary circles in the air from about a foot away.

Take note of the proximity where you may begin to notice the aroma. This denotes the *aroma strength*. Hold the strip close to your nose, breathe in briskly, and after take gradual and deep inhalations.

● **Step-3:** At this stage, start to take down notes. Denote the aroma with whatever words you may describe to it. It could be emotions, thoughts, images, sounds, colors, textures, shapes, etc.

● **Step-4:** Take a break and allow the essential oil to evaporate for about 10-30 minutes. Clear the palates in your nose by sniffing some fresh coffee grounds.

Go back to smell the strip. Take notes again, whether the initial aroma lasted a long time, or if it was light or heavy. Attach terms like green, floral, fruity, and mossy to describe the fragrance. Identify the principal trait of the note, whether it is musky, grassy, or nutty.

● **Step-5:** Liberate your imaginations. Envision the aroma as a shape, whether it is tiny, large, boxy, round, rough, level, or sharp.

● **Step-6:** Imagine the aroma with a personality. Close your eyes and describe the association, whether it is charismatic, shy, seductive, spunky, passionate, or friendly.

💧 **Step-7:** Be mindful of your body by observing your physical and emotional feelings, whether the essential oil is volatile, traveled straight to your chest, or darted quickly into your nose and between your eyes. Focus and further observe where in your inner spirit and body you feel the essential oil.

💧 **Step-8:** Finally, identify and distinguish your five selected oils into the categorical notes. The ideal results will have, at least, 2-top notes, 2-middle notes, and 1-base note.

💧 Picking the Perfect Pair:

Still, with your chosen five essential oils, it is critical to consider the strengths of their aromas when blending your oils. Be careful not to confuse *aroma strength* with the *rate of evaporation,* which is the measure of how fast the aroma evaporates from the strip.

Never blend powerful aromas in equal quantities for a formula, otherwise, it will overpower the blend, making an imbalanced blend. For example, take a blend of Roman chamomile oil and lavender oil.

Note that Roman chamomile oil has a stronger aroma than lavender oil. Thus, you will need more lavender oil to compensate a balanced blend; else, the aroma of the Roman chamomile dominates the blend.

To complement both aromas of Roman chamomile and lavender oils, you need to blend one drop of Roman chamomile to 4-8 drops of lavender. Now, this may catch you by surprise. **How will you know the proper ratios to blend?**

⬥ Rendering the Right Ratios:

Blending ratios are not works of magic, but you can determine them by creating your *aroma wand:* prepare 5 separate strips, one each for your chosen 5 essential oils, and place a few drops of the oils on one end of their designated strip. Create a fan out of these strips by holding their untainted ends with your thumb and forefinger so that you can waft the strips back and forth close to your nose while inhaling them.

This becomes a critical moment when adjusting the blending ratios based on *aroma strength*. A reliable rule of thumb is to begin deriving your aromatherapy blending formula on 100-drops so that it will be easier for you to determine the percentage of each essential oil in the blend.

You can decrease or increase the formula, provided you ensure to maintain the blending ratio. Always keep in mind that there is neither right nor wrong in rendering the ratios. This is your blend after all. If the formula does not quite satisfy your expectations, never be discouraged. Try again!

NOTE: Find positivity in your blending blunders. They can still be useful, perhaps, for cleaning! The bottom line is that nothing must go to waste.

When you are unsure where to get rolling, or are having difficulties in determining the notes, fragrances, or ratio ideas, take a break and your own sweet time. Review the following samples of pre-formulated essential oil blends (refer to Image-5).

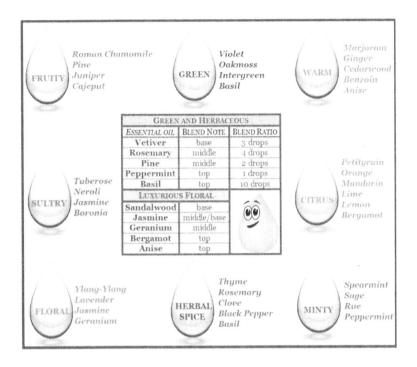

Image-5: Fragrance, Notes & Ratio Ideas

This will give you a guided idea on your personal preferences when blending your essential oils. Refer to Chapter-3 for more oils that you may like to blend.

Always remember to be mindful while you are formulating. Pause, breathe in, and allow the aroma and your senses to lead you towards your next choice.

You can blend different oils together to achieve a synergy, meaning you will be able enjoy the best of all the oils' worlds. Their respective natural powers will alter, enhancing their energies into one. Upon reaching a certain level of power, you have achieved a synergy!

ESSENTIAL OIL VS CARRIER OIL

Once you have finally chosen your preferred essential oil, they can be added to your health and beauty products to enhance the functionalities of these items. This means you dilute your oils to unscented hand and body lotions, bath oils, shower gels, and massage lotions.

Since essential oils are extremely volatile and sensitive to light, their healing aromas can evaporate quickly before they could serve your indentations of using them. You certainly would not like to waste their inherent energies or powers when applying them *neat-on,* or undiluted.

Therefore, NEVER apply essential oils directly to any surface of your skin. Instead, ALWAYS dilute them in water, a base oil, or carrier oil.

Besides, when applied to your skin undiluted, most essential oils, their *absolutes,* CO_2's (or *concretes* or *denatured* oils produced by solvent extraction), and other concentrated aromatics can trigger severe irritation, burning or redness, sensitizations, or other unwanted reactions.

You ought to use carrier oils to dilute the essential, and other, oils before applying them topically. Carrier oils derive their terminology from their main purpose of *carrying* essential oils onto the skin.

The noted Aloe Vera gel- and similarly unscented natural lotions, body oils, creams, lip balms, bath oils, and other moisturizing beauty and skin care products- are referred to as *carriers*. However, for the scope of this book, we will be focusing on the application of natural vegetable oils as carrier oils.

Generally, carrier oils come from the fatty sections of a plant. They primarily help maintain the intrinsic aroma of essential oils for a longer duration.

They provide a different combination of therapeutic characteristics and properties. Hence, your preference of carrier oils depends upon the therapeutic benefits you are seeking.

In addition, from a basic dilution of an essential oil and carrier oil resulting in a more complex natural blend, your choice of carrier oil can lead to a difference in color and overall aroma, as well as shelf life and potent effects of your final blended product. The following is a list of profiles of carrier oils commonly used in aromatherapy to help you choose. (refer to Image-6).

CARRIER OIL	LATIN NAME	AROMA	VISCOSITY	FEEL/ABSORPTION	COLOR	SHELF LIFE
Apricot (Kernel)	Prunus armeniaca	faint	light to medium	absorbs fast	clear with yellow tinge	1 to 2-years
Avocado	Persea americana	sweet, fatty, nutty	thick	leaves a fatty, waxy feel	deep olive green	12-months
Borage (Seed)	Borago officinalis	light, sweet	thin to medium	absorbs well, leaves oily film on skin	light yellow	6-months
Camellia Seed (Tea Oil)	Camellia oleifera	light	medium		pale to golden yellow	1-2 years
Coconut (Fractionated)	Cocos nucifera	odorless	light	non-greasy, absorbs well	clear	highly stable
Coconut (Virgin)	Cocos nucifera	very fragrant coconut	creamy at room temp.	slight oily feeling upon application	white	highly stable
Cranberry (Seed)	Vaccinium macrocarpon	fruity, bitter, but pleasant	medium		golden yellow	2 years
Evening Primrose	Oenothera biennis	light, sweet	thin	leaves traces of oil on skin	medium yellow	6-months
Grapeseed	Vitus vinifera	light, sweet slightly nutty	thin	leaves glossy film on skin	clear, tinge of yellow/green	6-12 months
Hazelnut	Corylus avellana	light, nutty, sweet	thin	leaves slight oily film on skin	light yellow	12 months
Hemp (Seed)	Cannabis sativa	faint, slightly nutty	medium		light to medium green	6-12 months
Jojoba	Simmondsia chinensis	light-medium, pleasant	medium	absorbs well	golden yellow	highly stable
Kukui (Nut)	Aleurites moluccana	light, pleasant, nutty, sweet	thin	absorbs well, leaves slight oily film on skin	clear with yellow tinge	12 months
Macadamia (Nut)	Macadamia integrifolia	sweet, nutty, fragrant nut	thick	leaves oily film on skin	clear with yellow tinge	12 months
Meadowfoam	Limnanthes alba	odorless	medium	penetrates well	pale yellow	highly stable
Olive	Olea europaea	fruity, slightly peppery	thick	oily	light to medium green	1-2 years
Peanut	Arachis hypogeae	light, nutty, fatty	thick	leaves a heavy, oily film on skin	clear	12 months
Pecan	Carya pecan	light, nutty	medium	absorbs well, leaves oily film on skin	clear	12 months
Pomegranate (Seed)	Punica granatum	odorless	medium	light and absorbs well	yellow	12 months
Rose Hip	Rosa mosqueta	mild, slightly earthy	light	leaves hints of oil on the ski	clear	6-12 months
Seabuckthorn (Berry)	Hippophae rhamnoides		medium	oily feel, for dilution to approx. 1%	seed oil—yellow pulp oil—orange	12 months
Sesame	Sesamum indicum	faint, sweet, nutty sesame	medium-thick	leaves oily film on the skin	pale yellow	12 months
Sunflower	Helianthus annuus	faint, sweet	thin	absorbs well, no traces of oily residue	clear with yellow tinge	12 months
Sweet Almond	Prunus amygdalus var. dulcus	light, sweet, nutty	medium	absorbs fast	clear with yellow tinge	1 to 2-years
Watermelon (Seed)	Citrullus vulgaris	faint, slightly, nutty	light	absorbs well	yellow	indefinite highly stable

Image-6: Aromatherapy Carrier Oils Profiles

Generally regarded as best and safest carrier oils for dilution—even for toddlers and children—are Jojoba, Sweet Almond, and Grapeseed oils. Apricot kernel and coconut oils are also better options for adults.

You may use olive oil, but its strong peppery scent may influence the blend. This is one principal reason it is not a regular oil fixture in aromatherapy.

DILUTION DO'S AND DON'TS:

You simply need to follow the recipes of your blending processes to attain an optimal synergy. However, you should leave your oils to age for a minimum of a week prior to diluting them to any base or carrier oils.

Your guide for diluting oils in accordance with specific applications/applicants are (refer to Images-7 & 8):

APPLICATION	RECOMMENDED DILUTION PROPORTION (ESSENTIAL OIL DROPS TO UNIT CARRIER OIL)
MASSAGE	5-drops per 1-tsp of lotion or base oil
INHALATION	1 or 2-drops in boiling water or on a cotton ball or tissue
BATH	6-drops in ¼-cup carrier oil; add 10-drops of blend to bath
SAUNA	2-drops to 2 ½-cups water
FACIAL	2 or 3-drops in base product
FOOT BATH	8-drops in bowl of water
FACIAL SAUNA	10-drops in bowl of water
CLEANSER	20-drops in 4-oz. of base product
BODY	5 to 15-drops in base product
CHEST RUB	10 to 20-drops to 1-oz. of carrier oil
LAUNDRY WASH	10 to 20-drops per laundry load
VACUUM CLEANER	5 to 10-drops
AUTO VENT OUTLET	2 or 3-drops
ARTIFICIAL HOLIDAY TREE	10 to 15-drops in 8-oz. of water

Image-7: Ideal Dilution Ratios per Application

Single Oil Name	Adult	Children	Pregnant	Commercial Oil Blend Name	Adult	Children	Pregnant
Basil	N	1:1	A	Aroma Touch	N	N	N
Bergamot	N**	N**	N**	Balance	N	N	N
Birch	N	1:1	A	Breathe	N	1:1	N
Cassie	1:4	C	A	Citrus Bliss	N*	N*	N*
Chamomile	N	1:1	N	Clear Skin Topical	N	N	C
Cinnamon	1:3	C	A	Deep Blue	N	1:1	N
Clary sage	N	N	C	Digest Zen	N	N	C
Clove	1:1	1:4	C	Elevation	N*	N*	N*
Coriander	N	N	N	Immortelle	N	N	C
Cypress	N	N	C	On Guard	N	1:1	C
Eucalyptus	N	1:1	N	Past Tense	N	1:1	C
Fennel	N	1:1	C	Purify	N	N	N
Frankincense	N	N	N	Serenity	N	N	N
Geranium	N	1:1	N	Slim & Sassy	N	1:1*	N
Ginger	N*	1:1	N	Solace	N	1:1	N
Grapefruit	N	N	N	Terra Shield	N	N	N
Helichrysum	N	N	N	Whisper	N	N	N
Lavender	N	N	N	Zendocrine	1:1	1:4	C
Lemon	N*	N*	N*	**LEGEND**			
Lemongrass	N	1:1	1:1	**N** ⇨ Can be used neat or without dilution			
Lime	N*	1:1	N*				
Marjoram	N	1:1	C	**C** ⇨ use with extreme caution; dilute heavily			
Melissa	N	N	N				
Myrrh	N	N	N	**A** ⇨ avoid using			
Orange	N*	N*	N*	**1:1** ⇨ Proportional ratio of essential oil (1st digit) to carrier oil (2nd digit) for dilution prior to applying			
Patchouli	N	N	N				
Peppermint	N	1:1	C				
Rose	N	N	N	**Photosensitivity Levels:**			
Rosemary	N	C	A	* ⇨ Avoid sunlight 12 hrs. after use			
Sandalwood	N	C	N	** ⇨ Avoid sunlight 12 hrs. after use			
Ylang-ylang	N	N	N				

Image-8: Essential Oil Dilution Chart

When having extremely sensitive skin, especially with children, it is crucially fundamental to test a small area of the skin before using any single essential oil or blend. Alternatively, you should also perform a skin-patch evaluation prior to your initial application to test for any irritation or potential allergic reactions. To execute:

♦ **Skin-Patch Test:** Apply a small amount of a diluted essential oil to the inside part of your elbow or forearm. Immediately cover the area with a patch or bandage. Observe for 24 hours to see whether any irritation occurs. If you do not experience any adverse reaction like swelling or itching, then the diluted oil should be safe for application elsewhere.

Safekeeping & Storage

It is no secret that some essential oils can fetch a steeper price than thought. For rarer types, a single tablespoon or half an ounce may cost well over $50! Perhaps that is tolerable or just a pittance for some.

Nonetheless, the worst part is that essential oils spoil easily. Any essential oil, regardless of having a longer shelf life, can spoil within just a week after being subjected or exposed to light, heat, moisture, or oxygen. You can just imagine the loss!

An exposure to any of these elements results in oxidation, which quickly sets off the process of evaporation. Just the same, while essential oils do not typically become rancid, they still oxidize.

Through the process of oxidation, each essential oil alters its physical structure and chemical composition, thus reducing or losing its beneficial therapeutic qualities over the passage of time. In particular, citrus oils easily oxidize and can start losing their aromas and healing powers in as little as six months.

However, not all essential oils deteriorate in aromatic quality over time. The aromas of sandalwood and patchouli typically mature with age.

Categorized by the National Fire Protection Association (NFPA) as Class-3 Flammable Liquids, most essential oils are relatively combustible with *flashpoints* (lowest temperatures at which they ignite) ranging between 122°F to 140°F (50°C to 60°C). Light and heat increase your oils' latent temperature, which might cause them to break down and burn.

Light energy, particularly sunlight, is notorious for altering the color of essential oils as time goes by. Besides being highly volatile, essential oils can easily alter its state with the existences of new energy like light or heat.

Therefore, to avoid deterioration and maintain a longer viability of the therapeutic and aromatic properties of your oils right after purchasing them, they ought to be stored safely and protected accordingly.

All essential oils, as well as you, will certainly benefit from proper handling and storage. Here are a dozen handling methods and storage techniques you should implement to maximize the shelf life of your aromatherapy oils:

💧 Do not keep your oils anywhere and expect them to continue doing wonders to you and your life. Keep all your bottled oils away from a humid atmosphere. Instead, store them inside cool, dark, and dry places.

💧 For some essential oils, as well as your carrier oils, the refrigerator is their ideal sanctuary. You can always take out your carrier oils from the fridge 12 hours prior to using them. Just warm them slightly with your palms.

◆ To shield your oils from exposures to light, store them in green, cobalt, blue, or amber-colored glass bottles instead of clear or transparent ones. Colored glasses can block the sun's ultraviolet rays in the same manner as beer bottled in amber-colored bottled does. Transparent containers simply allow the transmission of light liberally.

◆ Never place your oil bottles on the windowsills or in areas adjacent to open windows that let in sunlight.

◆ Keep your oil bottles away from imminent sources of flames and ignitions like fires and stoves.

◆ Never allow the build-up of space in your oil containers. Always keep your oil containers full by transferring your oils from large and half-empty containers to smaller ones. The principle behind this is to reduce the airspace inside your container to limit risks of oxidation.

◆ After using an essential oil, always ensure closing the bottle immediately to prevent entry of oxygen.

♦ Never store your oils inside plastic bottles. The oils will corrode the container and degrade it completely.

♦ Keep your oil bottles away from the reach of curious little hands.

♦ Some merchants sell oils in aluminum-lined bottles. Aluminum bottles are acceptable as long as there is a lining inside.

♦ A rubber dropper is prone to mixing with your pure oil or melting away over time. Avoid using them.

♦ Always keep the orifice reducer in place in the bottle since it also helps with sealing.

Safety Standards

Although using essential oils may have endless lists of benefits, you still need to exercise extra care and caution to avoid hazards and chronic side effects like rashes, allergies, headaches, and even death. The following are the most urgent safety reminders to bear in mind when using essential oils:

● Always dilute your essential oils with carrier oils prior to applying on your skin to avoid irritation, burning, and other side effects.

● Always check the label of the packaging or bottle for noting the oil's dilution and preparation guidelines before using it. If you find none, then consult with a certified aromatherapist.

● Perform a *skin-patch test* for each of the different oils before you apply them to your body.

● For children, essential oils are not advised or necessary as part of their bath. These cherubs still have sensitive skins that require extreme care.

● Do not allow children, aged 7 years old and below, to inhale essential oils from a heated or steamed solution. For children over 7 years old, they should wear the necessary safety goggles during the process.

● Keep your essential oils out of reach of pets, pests, and children to avoid wastage and accidents.

♦ Never bathe in water blended with essential oils without first putting in a dispersant, like Epsom salts. Essential oils do not dissolve in water sans a dispersant; thus, your blended bath water becomes hazardous for use without it.

♦ Avoid the application of essential oils to the different sensitive parts of your body like the eyes, mouth, ears, and genitals. If it is necessary for you to apply, then strictly follow the dilution guidelines to prevent irritations of the sensitive skin.

♦ All citrus oils, including their derivatives, can make your skin more sensitive to ultraviolet light. Never expose your skin to the sun while using these oils.

♦ Always prefer the high-quality essential oils from trusted brands and retailers to avoid adulterated oils or added flavorings, synthetic chemicals, and fragrances that might activate allergies and harmful side effects.

Further medical research has contributed other specific safety measures to follow for the proper application of essential oils. The stipulations made by the University of Maryland Medical Center include:

◆ Pregnant women and nursing or breastfeeding mothers must avoid essential oils.

◆ Individuals with medical histories of allergies and severe asthma should only use the aromatic oils under the proper guidance of a skilled professional or the full consent and knowledge of their physician.

◆ Individuals receiving chemotherapy treatments should consult with their physician before engaging with aromatherapy.

◆ Individuals with medical histories of epilepsy or seizures should avoid using rosemary, sage, fennel, and hyssop oils. These oils have *nervine* (nerve-stimulating) properties that could trigger recurrence and aggravate the condition

◆ Individuals with estrogen-dependent cysts or tumors like ovarian or breast cancer should not use clary sage, Spanish sage, aniseed, and fennel oils, which have estrogen-like compounds.

⧫ Individuals with high blood pressure should avoid using basil, eucalyptus, rosemary, patchouli, and mint oils, which are highly stimulating essential oils.

⧫ NEVER ingest essential oils. Aromatherapy oils and its techniques do not intend to diagnose, treat, or prevent any illnesses. It is only a natural supplement to equilibrate and augment the healing process.

Similar to trying any new medical treatment, ALWAYS seek the consultation of a trained aromatherapist or your doctor before using essential oils or engaging with aromatherapy. Your medical history is significant for giving you the green light to venture further in to aromatherapy.

In conclusion, these safety tips are as vital as the countless benefits of essential oils. Aromatherapy remains incomplete and useless without gaining the benefits of the essential oils; more so, on learning their application guidelines and safety measures.

Procurement Practices

With numerous essential oils, *absolutes*, *denatured CO_2's*, and *hydrosols* available in the market today, it can be a confusing and daunting experience, especially for beginners, to purchase the right, and quality, essential oils best suited for one's specific needs and budget. However, you should only keep in mind some important factors and parameters on the proper ways of buying your essential oils.

PURCHASING PARAMETERS

To begin with, pick essential oils that are stimulating, like rosemary and peppermint, and those that are calming, like chamomile and lavender. Generally, these twin principal properties of essential oils are mostly what you need to resolve many issues for your daily living and well-being.

For your proper guidance, here are the top 10 primary essential oils to start and fill your personal care kit:

- **Rosemary** – for promoting healthy blood circulation and overall wellness

- **Peppermint** – for promoting digestive health

- **Marjoram** – for promoting overall health and wellness

- **Lavender** – for promoting mood, relaxation, and overall wellness

- **Geranium** – for promoting balance of the mind and body

- **Eucalyptus** – for promoting skin and respiratory health

- **Cypress** – for promoting a healthy circulatory system and overall wellness

- **Chamomile (Roman/German)** – for promoting relaxation and digestive health and relaxation

- **Bergamot** – for promoting healthier moods and overall wellness

You can use them separately or in combination to concoct your own personalized blend. Having these primary oils, you can create several blends according to your needs.

As a precaution, know that additives are predominantly featured in many essential oils sold commercially today. Simply because the bottle states *100%-pure,* does not conclusively mean the essential oil is.

Many aromatherapy oil products sold in supermarkets do not really contain pure essential oils. They mostly have dilutions of synthetic fillers and chemicals, suspenders, or added vegetable and mineral oils that diminish their purity.

High quality and pure essential oils are unadulterated. You should read the label and ingredient contents of any aromatherapy oil you wish to buy

Additionally, purchase essential oils certified as organic on their labels. The packaging label may further mark the essential oil as either food-grade or therapeutic-grade. Prefer the therapeutic grade items.

⚫ **Food-Grade Essential Oils** – are usual mixtures of other synthetic chemicals before they reach the display stands, thus they cannot be more effective for aromatherapy use.

⚫ **Therapeutic-Grade Essential Oils** – are ideally the appropriate oils for your aromatherapy applications. Usually, their labels include displaying the Latin name of the essential oil's mother plant.

Still, these are not guaranteed for procuring high-quality oils, much less a high price on their tags. Please note that the U.S. Food and Drug Administration (FDA) does not regulate the entire industry of aromatherapy. Although some traders may have the approval certificates or regulated standards issued by the FDA, regardless not every brand or product you see in store or online, can be trustworthy.

This also denotes that you have to be more responsible by doing research about a particular essential oil product to be sure of its quality. It is advisable that you perform some background checks on the outfit selling aromatherapy essential oils.

To maximize your results, check the oil's origin and production processes—plant species, farming location, growing season and weather, harvesting methods, form of extraction, etc. These are only a few significant factors that define high-grade essential oils.

PEGGED PRICES

For personal use, it is common to find essential oils, *absolutes*, and *denatured CO_2's* sold in 5-mL, 10-mL and 15-mL (½-oz.) sizes. For rarer and more expensive oils, they can be available from 2-mL to 1-mL Avoirdupois dram sizes.

The prevailing market prices of each personal essential oil vary, starting from $10 or less to come costing more than $400 per 1-fluid ounce. Typically, the cost of essential oils are in direct proportion to the required quantities of raw plant material used to produce the oil.

For instance, oil extractors require 2,000-pounds, or 1-ton, of the rose's flower petals to produce only a single pound of rose essential oil. This would seem like liquid gold, and easily fetching up a high selling price! In stark comparison, oil extractors only require 50-pounds of a eucalyptus raw plant material to produce the same quantity of eucalyptus essential oil.

Tools of the Trade

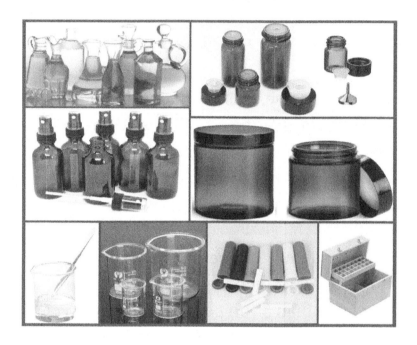

Image-9: Essential Oil Blending Kit Essentials

TOP ROW: *Carriers, Amber Bottles with Caps and Orifice Reducers*
MIDDLE ROW: *Amber Glass Spray Bottles, Amber Glass Jars*
BOTTOM ROW: *Mixing Glass with Spout and Glass Stirring Rod, Beakers, Blank Nasal Inhalers, and Essential Oil Blending Kit*

The fun and exciting world of aromatherapy and essential oils will soon let you discover that it can be truly overwhelming. It can be confusing how to determine what you need first and should buy immediately, or what things can be deferrable or wait for the meantime:

- Aromatic Room Spray
- Body Lotion and Facial Cream
- Bottle Spray
- Massage Oil or Liniment
- Liquid Hand Soap
- Nasal Inhaler
- Salt Scrub
- Diffuser, which comes as several types such as atomizing/nebulizer, ultrasonic/humidifying, electric heat, evaporative, fan-style, terracotta and sandstone, candle/aromatherapy lamp

To simplify and help you to avoid useless purchases you do not immediately need, here is a basic list from which you can start engaging with aromatherapy.

ESSENTIAL EQUIPMENT FOR BLENDING BASICS

⬥ **Essential Oils:** To begin a more modest investment, purchase your essential oils packaged in 5-mL bottles. Prefer the top 10 list of primary essential oils mentioned previously in the section, <u>Purchasing Parameters</u>. The chamomiles will be the most costly.

⬥ **Carrier Oils:** As the foundation for most of your blends to dilute oils so they can be applicable to the skin, have a supply of the basic carriers:

- ✓ 8-oz. Unscented Lotion
- ✓ 16-oz. Jojoba Oil
- ✓ 16-oz. Pink Himalayan Salt
- ✓ 16-oz. Liquid Castile Soap

⬥ **Containers:** You will need jars and bottles in which to use or store your blend.

- ✓ 2-oz. or 4-oz. glass spray bottle
- ✓ 2-oz. glass jars with lids for lotions
- ✓ 5-mL, 10-mL or 15-mL amber glass bottles with caps and orifice reducer

- **Glassware for Blending with Glass Stir Rod:** These are convenient receptacles where you can blend your oils and carriers effortlessly- besides, they are easy to clean.

- **Measuring Cups or Glass Beakers:** Although beakers are a little expensive, they are worth it for their significant functions for blending. For convenience, you need 5-mL, 10-mL, 25-mL, and 50-mL sizes.

- **Blank Nasal Inhaler:** It is advisable that you begin with a pack of 10 pieces. Prefer the colored ones for easy identification of the blends.

- **Miscellaneous:**

  ✓ Waterproof Markers and Labels – for marking a clever name for your blend, its blending date, ratio or drop proportions, ingredients, and any significant notes you want to remember. Your markers should be waterproof to avoid ink smudges. Mailing sizes are ideal for your labels.
  ✓ Microfiber Towels or Paper Towels for wiping spills
  ✓ Cotton Balls or Tissue Paper for inhaling
  ✓ Journal/Notebook for recording your recipe blends

⬥ **Blending Kit:** If you do not have any space to store your tools and blends, then you can purchase some wooden aromatherapy blending kit. It keeps all your aromatherapy equipment and items together in one place.

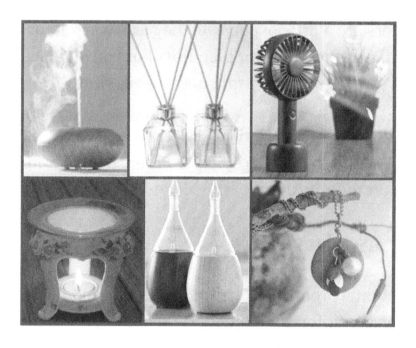

Image-10: Types of Essential Oil Diffuser

TOP ROW: Ultrasonic or Humidifying, Evaporative, and Fan-Type
BOTTOM ROW: Aromatherapy Lamp with Tea Candlelight, Nebulizer or Atomizing, Terracotta and Sandstone Necklace

Chapter 3 - Nature's Nourishments

Aromatherapy sources a large number of its scents from the apothecary of nature. Mostly, they come from fragrant flowers, healthy herbs and a few from shrubs and trees.

With so many of them, it can be perplexing which aromatic essential oils are most suitable for aromatherapy and which are not. Remember, not all essential oils are equal. Some are highly toxic and not fit for aromatherapy practices.

The following is a comprehensive and informative list that serves as your quick guide to 100 neatly detailed essential oils that are satisfactorily acceptable for aromatherapy. This exclusive list, alphabetically organized, will help you easily to find which aromatic essential oils will benefit you most in accordance to your needs.

Fragrant Flowers | Healthy Herbs: Aromatherapy Aromas

1-ALLSPICE

💧 **Attached Latin name:** *Pimenta dioica*

💧 **Applications:** circulatory system—arthritis, fatigue, muscle cramp, rheumatism, stiffness, etc. | respiratory system—chills, congestion, bronchitis | digestive system—cramp, flatulence, indigestion, nausea | nervous system—depression, nervous exhaustion, neuralgia, tension, stress | in small amounts, massage oil for chest infections

💧 **Attributes:** anesthetic, analgesic, antioxidant, antiseptic, carminative, muscle relaxant, rubefacient, stimulant, and tonic

💧 **Aroma:** leaf oil—a similar fragrance to cloves | berry oil—sweet, warm balsamic-spicy body note, fresh clean top note

💧 **Ably blends with:** ginger, geranium, lavender, labdanum, ylang-ylang, patchouli, neroli, Oriental, and spicy bases

💧 **Abundant areas:** indigenous to the West Indies, South America, cultivated in Jamaica and Cuba

* **Acquisition:** steam distillation of the leaves and fruit
* **Areas of safety:** cause dermal irritation due to eugenol contents, which irritate mucous membranes, use in low dilutions only

2-AMBRETTE SEED

* **Attached Latin name:** *Abelmoschus moschatus*
* **Applications:** circulation system—cramp, fatigue, muscular aches and pains, poor circulation | nervous system—anxiety, depression, nervous tension and stress related conditions
* **Attributes:** antispasmodic, aphrodisiac, carminative, nervine, stimulant, and stomachic
* **Aroma:** tenaciously sweet, floral-musky
* **Ably blends with:** roses, neroli, sandalwood, clary sage, cypress, patchouli, Oriental and sophisticated bases
* **Abundant areas:** native to India, cultivated in tropical countries like Indonesia, Africa, Egypt, China, Madagascar, and West Indies
* **Acquisition:** steam distillation of seeds | absolute & concrete produced by solvent extraction

♦ **Areas of safety:** non-toxic, non-irritant, and non-sensitizing

3-ANGELICA

♦ **Attached Latin name:** *Angelica archangelica*

♦ **Applications:** skin care, psoriasis, arthritis, gout, rheumatism, water retention, bronchitis, coughs, anemia, anorexia, flatulence, indigestion, fatigue, migraine, nervous tension, stress-related disorders, colds

♦ **Attributes:** antispasmodic, carminative, depurative, diaphoretic, digestive, diuretic, emmenagogue, expectorant, febrifuge, nervine, stimulant, stomachic, and tonic

♦ **Aroma:** rich herbaceous body note while the seed oil has a fresher spicy top note

♦ **Ably blends with:** patchouli, costus, clary sage, oakmoss, vetiver, and citrus oils

♦ **Abundant areas:** native to Europe and Siberia, cultivated in Belgium, Hungary, and Germany

♦ **Acquisition:** steam distillation of roots, rhizomes, and fruits/seeds | absolute—produced on a small scale from the roots by solvent extraction

- **Areas of safety:** non-toxic and non-irritant | not used during pregnancy or by diabetics

4-ANISE

- **Attached Latin name:** *Pimpinella anisum*
- **Applications:** muscular aches and pains, rheumatism, bronchitis, coughs, colic, cramp, flatulence, indigestion, colds
- **Attributes:** antiseptic, carminative, expectorant, insect repellent, stimulant
- **Aroma:** warm, spicy, extremely sweet, licorice-like scent
- **Ably blends with:** rose, lavender, orange, pine, and other spice oils
- **Abundant areas:** native to South East China, Vietnam, India, and Japan
- **Acquisition:** steam distillation of fruits, fresh or partially dried | leaves can produce oil in small quantities
- **Areas of safety:** does not appear to be a dermal irritant | narcotic in large doses and slows down circulation that can lead to cerebral disorders | use in moderation

5-Arnica

♦ **Attached Latin name:** *Arnica montana*
♦ **Applications:** asthma, bronchitis, whooping cough, fatigue, nervous exhaustion, stress-related conditions
♦ **Attributes:** antispasmodic, carminative, expectorant, hypotensive, stimulant
♦ **Aroma:** tenacious odor resembling garlic; beneath is a sweet, balsamic note
♦ **Ably blends with:** no available data
♦ **Abundant areas:** native to Afghanistan, Iran, and other regions of Southwest Asia
♦ **Acquisition:** steam distillation of the oleoresin obtained by making incisions into the root and above ground parts of the plant, the milky juice left to leak out, and harden | steam distillation also produces absolute, tincture, and resinous substances
♦ **Areas of safety:** non-toxic and non-irritant in its pure form

6-Balm (Lemon)

♦ **Attached Latin name:** *Melissa officinalis*

◆ **Applications:** allergies, insect bites, insect repellent, eczema, asthma, bronchitis, chronic coughs, colic, indigestion, nausea, menstrual problems, anxiety, depression, hypertension, insomnia, migraine, nervous tension, shock, and vertigo

◆ **Attributes:** antidepressant, antihistaminic, antispasmodic, bactericidal, carminative, cordial, diaphoretic, emmenagogue, febrifuge, hypertensive, insect repellent, nervine, sedative, stomachic, sudorific, tonic, uterine, and vermifuge

◆ **Aroma:** light, fresh, and lemony

◆ **Ably blends with:** lavender, geranium, floral and citrus oils

◆ **Abundant areas:** native to the Mediterranean, cultivated in France, Spain, Germany and Russia, common throughout Europe, Middle Asia, North America, North Africa, and Siberia

◆ **Acquisition:** steam distillation of leaves and flowering tops

◆ **Areas of safety:** non-toxic, but may cause sensitivity and dermal irritation | use in low dilutions only

7-BALSAM (CANADIAN)

- **Attached Latin name:** *Abies balsamea*
- **Applications:** burns, cuts, hemorrhoids, wounds, asthma, bronchitis, catarrh, chronic coughs, sore throat, cystitis, genital-urinary infections, depression, nervous tension, stress related conditions
- **Attributes:** antiseptic (genital-urinary, pulmonary) antitussive, astringent, cicatrizant, diuretic, expectorant, purgative, regulatory, sedative (nerve), tonic, and vulnerary
- **Aroma:** fresh, sweet, balsamic, almost fruity
- **Ably blends with:** pine, cedarwood, cypress, sandalwood, juniper, benzoin, and other balsams
- **Abundant areas:** native to North America Quebec, Nova Scotia, and Maine
- **Acquisition:** oleoresin collected by puncturing vesicles in the bark | steam distillation of the oleoresin
- **Areas of safety:** non-toxic, non-irritant, and non-sensitizing | do not use in large doses

8-BALSAM (COPAIBA)

- **Attached Latin name:** *Copaifera reticulata*

◆ **Applications:** intestinal infections, piles, bronchitis, chills, colds, coughs, cystitis, and stress-related conditions

◆ **Attributes:** bactericidal, balsamic, disinfectant, diuretic, expectorant, stimulant

◆ **Aroma:** crude balsam—hardens on exposure to air, mild, woody, slightly spicy odor | oil – mild, sweet, balsamic, and peppery

◆ **Ably blends with:** balsam—lavandin, cedarwood, lavender, oakmoss, woods, and spices | oil –ylang-ylang, jasmine, and other florals

◆ **Abundant areas:** native to Northeast and Central South America, produced in Brazil, Venezuela, Guyana, Surinam, and Columbia

◆ **Acquisition:** dry distillation of the crude balsam

◆ **Areas of safety:** non-toxic and non-irritant, but may cause sensitivity | large doses cause vomiting and diarrhea

9-BALSAM (PERU)

◆ **Attached Latin name:** *Myroxylon balsamum*

♦ **Applications:** dry, chapped skin, eczema, rashes, sores, sounds, low blood pressure, rheumatism, asthma, bronchitis, coughs, colds, nervous tension, and stress

♦ **Attributes:** anti-inflammatory, antiseptic, antiparasitic, balsamic, expectorant, stimulant, promotes the growth of epithelial cells

♦ **Aroma:** rich, sweet, balsamic, vanilla-like

♦ **Ably blends with:** ylang-ylang, patchouli, petitgrain, sandalwood, rose, spices, floral, and Oriental bases

♦ **Abundant areas:** native to Central America, produced in El Salvador

♦ **Acquisition:** high vacuum dry distillation of crude balsam

♦ **Areas of safety:** oil—non-toxic and non-irritant | balsam—a common contact allergen, which may cause dermatitis

10-BASIL

♦ **Attached Latin name:** *Ocimum basilicum*

♦ **Applications:** insect bites, insect repellent, gout, muscular aches and pains, rheumatism, bronchitis, coughs, earache, sinusitis, dyspepsia, flatulence, nausea, cramps, scanty periods, colds, fever, flu, and infectious diseases

♦ **Attributes:** antidepressant, antiseptic, antispasmodic, carminative, cephalic, digestive, emmenagogue, expectorant, febrifuge, galactagogic, nervine, prophylactic, restorative, a stimulant of the adrenal cortex, stomachic, tonic.

♦ **Aroma:** light, fresh, sweet-spicy, and balsamic undertone

♦ **Ably blends with:** bergamot, clary sage, lime, oakmoss, citronella, geranium, hyssop, and other green notes

♦ **Abundant areas:** native to tropical Asia and Africa, cultivated in Europe, Mediterranean, Pacific Islands, North, and South America

♦ **Acquisition:** steam distillation of leaves

♦ **Areas of safety:** non-toxic and non-irritant, but may cause sensitivity in some | do not use during pregnancy

11-BAY LAUREL

♦ **Attached Latin name:** *Laurus nobilis*

♦ **Applications:** dyspepsia, flatulence, loss of appetite, scanty periods, colds, flu, tonsillitis, and viral infections

♦ **Attributes:** anti-rheumatic, antiseptic, bactericidal, diaphoretic, digestive, diuretic, emmenagogue, fungicidal, hypotensive, sedative, and stomachic

♦ **Aroma:** powerful, spicy-medicinal

♦ **Ably blends with:** pine, cypress, juniper, clary sage, rosemary, labdanum, lavender, citrus, and spice oils

♦ **Abundant areas:** native to the Mediterranean region; cultivated in France, Spain, Italy, Morocco, Yugoslavia, China, Israel, Turkey, and Russia

♦ **Acquisition:** steam distillation of leaves

♦ **Areas of safety:** non-toxic and non-irritant, but may cause dermatitis in some

12-BAY (WEST INDIAN)

♦ **Attached Latin name:** *Pimenta racemosa*

♦ **Applications:** scalp stimulant, hair rinse for dandruff, greasy, lifeless hair and promoting growth, muscular and articular aches and pains, neuralgia, poor circulation, rheumatism, sprains, strains, colds, flu, and infectious diseases

● **Attributes:** analgesic, anticonvulsant, anti-neuralgic, anti-rheumatic, antiseptic, astringent, expectorant, stimulant, tonic for hair

● **Aroma:** fresh-spicy top note and sweet balsamic undertone

● **Ably blends with:** lavender, lavandin, rosemary, geranium, ylang-ylang, citrus, and spice oils

● **Abundant areas:** native to the West Indies

● **Acquisition:** water or steam distillation of leaves

● **Areas of safety:** moderately toxic due to high eugenol content | a mucous membrane irritant | use in moderation

13. BENZOIN

● **Attached Latin name:** *Styrax benzoin*

● **Applications:** cuts, chapped skin, inflamed and irritated conditions, arthritis, gout, poor circulation, rheumatism, asthma, bronchitis, chills, colic, coughs, laryngitis, flu, nervous tension, and stress-related complaints

♦ **Attributes:** anti-inflammatory, anti-oxidant, antiseptic, astringent, carminative, cordial, deodorant, diuretic, expectorant, sedative, styptic, and vulnerary

♦ **Aroma:** intensely rich, sweet, and balsamic

♦ **Ably blends with:** sandalwood, roses, jasmine, copaiba balsam, frankincense, myrrh, cypress, juniper, lemon, coriander, and other spice oils

♦ **Abundant areas:** native to tropical Asia, Sumatra, Java, Malaysia, Laos, Vietnam, Cambodia, China, and Thailand

♦ **Acquisition:** crude benzoin collected directly from the trees and sold dissolved in ethyl glycol or similar solvent

♦ **Areas of safety:** non-toxic and non-irritant, but may cause sensitivity

14-BERGAMOT

♦ **Attached Latin name:** *Citrus bergamia*

♦ **Applications:** skin care, acne, boils, cold sores, eczema, insect repellent, insect bites, oily complexion, psoriasis, scabies, spots, varicose ulcers, wounds, halitosis, mouth infections, sore throat, tonsillitis, flatulence, loss of appetite, cystitis, leucorrhoea, itches, thrust, colds, fever, 'flu, infectious diseases, anxiety, depression, and stress-related conditions

♦ **Attributes:** analgesic, antihelmintic, antidepressant, antiseptic, antiparasitic, antispasmodic, antitoxic, carminative, digestive, diuretic, deodorant, febrifuge, laxative, rubefacient, stimulant, stomachic, tonic, vermifuge, and vulnerary

♦ **Aroma:** fresh, sweet-fruity, slightly spicy, and balsamic undertone

♦ **Ably blends with:** lavender, neroli, jasmine, cypress, geranium, lemon, chamomile, juniper, coriander, opopanax, and violet

♦ **Abundant areas:** native to tropical Asian regions, cultivated in Southern Italy and Ivory Coast

♦ **Acquisition:** cold expression of the peel of the nearly ripe fruit

♦ **Areas of safety:** non-toxic and non-irritant | sensitivity and skin pigmentation may occur when exposed to direct sunlight

15-BIRCH (WHITE)

♦ **Attached Latin name:** *Betula papyrifera*

♦ **Applications:** dermatitis, dull or congested skin, eczema, hair care, psoriasis, arthritis, cellulitis, muscular pain, obesity, edema, poor circulation, and rheumatism

♦ **Attributes:** anti-inflammatory, antiseptic, cholagogue, diaphoretic, diuretic, febrifuge, tonic

♦ **Aroma:** oil—woody, green, and balsamic | rectified oil—smoky and tar-like

♦ **Ably blends with:** other woody and balsamic oils

♦ **Abundant areas:** native to the Northern Hemisphere, Eastern Europe, Russia, Germany, Sweden, Finland, the Baltic coast, Northern China, and Japan

♦ **Acquisition:** steam distillation of leaves

♦ **Areas of safety:** non-toxic, non-irritant, and non-sensitivity

16-BORONIA (SYDNEY ROSE)

♦ **Attached Latin name:** *Boronia serrulata*
♦ **Applications:** perfume
♦ **Attributes:** aromatic
♦ **Aroma:** concrete—beautiful arm, woody-sweet fragrance | absolute—fresh, fruity-spicy scent with a rich tenacious floral undertone

💧 **Ably blends with:** clary sage, sandalwood, bergamot, violet, helichrysum, costus, mimosa, and other florals

💧 **Abundant areas:** native to Western Australia

💧 **Acquisition:** concrete and absolute—enfleurage method or petroleum-ether extraction | oil—a steam distillation of concrete produce small quantities

💧 **Areas of safety:** prohibitively expensive; and thus, often adulterated

17-CADE (CAJEPUT)

💧 **Attached Latin name:** *Melaleuca leucadendra*

💧 **Applications:** cuts, dandruff, dermatitis, eczema, and spots

💧 **Attributes:** analgesic, antimicrobial, antipruritic, antiseptic, anti-parasitic, disinfectant, and vermifuge

💧 **Aroma:** woody, smoky, and leather-like odor

💧 **Ably blends with:** clove, cassia, pine, and medicinal type bases

💧 **Abundant areas:** native to Southern France, Europe, and North Africa

💧 **Acquisition:** crude oil—destructive distillation | rectified oil—steam or vacuum distillation of crude oil | oil—a steam distillation of berries

♦ **Areas of safety:** non-toxic, non-irritant, but may cause sensitivity problems

18-CALAMINTHA

♦ **Attached Latin name:** *Clinopodium nepeta*
♦ **Applications:** chills, cold in the joints, muscular aches and pains, rheumatism, colic, flatulence, nervous dyspepsia, insomnia, nervous tension, and stress-related conditions
♦ **Attributes:** anesthetic, anti-rheumatic, antispasmodic, astringent, carminative, diaphoretic, emmenagogue, febrifuge, nervine, sedative, and tonic
♦ **Aroma:** herbaceous, woody, and pungent
♦ **Ably blends with:** no available data
♦ **Abundant areas:** native to Europe and parts of Asia; cultivated for oil in the Mediterranean region, Yugoslavia, Poland, and the USA
♦ **Acquisition:** steam distillation of leaves
♦ **Areas of safety:** non-irritant and non-sensitivity, but may cause toxic effects in concentration

19-CAMPHOR (WHITE)

♦ **Attached Latin name:** *Cinnamomum camphora*

💧 **Applications:** used with care for acne, inflammation, oil conditions, spots, insect prevention, arthritis, muscular aches and pains, rheumatism, sprains, bronchitis, chills, coughs, colds, fever, flu, and infectious diseases

💧 **Attributes:** anti-inflammatory, antiseptic, antiviral, bactericidal, counter-irritant, diuretic, expectorant, stimulant, rubefacient, and vermifuge

💧 **Aroma:** sharp, pungent, and camphoraceous

💧 **Ably blends with:** no data available

💧 **Abundant areas:** native to Japan and Taiwan, and China, cultivated in India, Ceylon, Egypt, Madagascar, Southern Europe, and America

💧 **Acquisition:** steam distillation of wood

💧 **Areas of safety:** white camphor—non-toxic, non-sensitizing, and non-irritant | brown/yellow camphor—toxic and carcinogenic, and not used in therapy, internally or externally

20-CARAWAY

💧 **Attached Latin name:** *Carum carvi*

💧 **Applications:** bronchitis, coughs, laryngitis, dyspepsia, colic, flatulence, gastric spasm, nervous indigestion, poor appetite, and colds

♦ **Attributes:** antihistaminic, antimicrobial, antiseptic, aperitif, astringent, carminative, diuretic, emmenagogue, expectorant, galactagogic, larvicidal, stimulant, spasmodic, stomachic, tonic, and vermifuge

♦ **Aroma:** oil—harsh and spicy | distilled oil—strong warm, sweet, and spicy

♦ **Ably blends with:** jasmine, cinnamon, and cassia

♦ **Abundant areas:** native to Europe and Western Asia, cultivated in Germany, Holland, Scandinavia, and Russia

♦ **Acquisition:** steam distillation of seeds

♦ **Areas of safety:** non-toxic and non-sensitivity, but may cause dermal irritation in concentration

21-CARDAMOM

♦ **Attached Latin name:** *Elettaria cardamomum*

♦ **Applications:** anorexia, colic, cramp, dyspepsia, flatulence, griping pains, halitosis, heartburn, indigestion, vomiting, mental fatigue, and nervous strain

♦ **Attributes:** antiseptic, antispasmodic, aphrodisiac, carminative, cephalic, digestive, diuretic, sialagogue, stimulant, stomachic, and tonic

◆ **Aroma:** sweet, spicy, and warm with a woody and balsamic undertone

◆ **Ably blends with:** roses, orange, bergamot, cinnamon, cloves, caraway, ylang-ylang, labdanum, cedarwood, neroli, and Oriental bases

◆ **Abundant areas:** native to tropical Asia and Southern India, cultivated in India, Sri Lanka, Laos, Guatemala, and El Salvador

◆ **Acquisition:** steam distillation of leaves

◆ **Areas of safety:** non-toxic, non-irritant, and non-sensitivity

22-CARROT SEED

◆ **Attached Latin name:** *Daucus carota*

◆ **Applications:** dermatitis, eczema, psoriasis, rashes, revitalizing and toning, mature complexions, wrinkles, arthritis, gout, edema, rheumatism, anemia, anorexia, colic, indigestion, liver congestion, amenorrhea, dysmenorrhea, glandular problems, and PMS

◆ **Attributes:** antihelmintic, antiseptic, carminative, depurative, diuretic, emmenagogue, hepatic, stimulant, tonic, vasodilatory, and smooth muscle relaxant

◆ **Aroma:** warm, dry, woody, and earthy

⚫ **Ably blends with:** costus, cassie, mimosa, cedarwood, geranium, citrus, and spice oils

⚫ **Abundant areas:** native to Europe, Asia, and North Africa

⚫ **Acquisition:** steam distillation of seeds

⚫ **Areas of safety:** non-toxic, non-irritant, and non-sensitivity

23-CASCARILLA

⚫ **Attached Latin name:** *Croton eluteria*

⚫ **Applications:** bronchitis, cough, dyspepsia, flatulence, nausea, and flu

⚫ **Attributes:** astringent, antimicrobial, antiseptic, carminative, digestive, expectorant, stomachic, and tonic

⚫ **Aroma:** spicy, warm, and woody

⚫ **Ably blends with:** nutmeg, pepper, sage, oakmoss, spicy, and Oriental bases

⚫ **Abundant areas:** native to the West Indies, grows wild in Mexico, Colombia, and Ecuador

⚫ **Acquisition:** steam distillation of leaves

⚫ **Areas of safety:** non-toxic, non-irritant, and non-sensitivity

24-Cassie

♦ **Attached Latin name:** *Vachellia tortuosa*

♦ **Applications:** used with care for dry, sensitive skin, perfume, depression, frigidity, nervous exhaustion, and stress-related conditions

♦ **Attributes:** anti-rheumatic, antiseptic, antispasmodic, aphrodisiac, balsamic, and insecticide

♦ **Aroma:** warm, floral, spicy

♦ **Ably blends with:** bergamot, costus, mimosa, frankincense, ylang-ylang, and violet

♦ **Abundant areas:** native to the West Indies, cultivated in tropical and semi-tropical regions of Southern France, Egypt, Lebanon, Morocco, Algeria, and India

♦ **Acquisition:** absolute—solvent extraction of flowers

♦ **Areas of safety:** no available data

25-Cedarwood (Atlas)

♦ **Attached Latin name:** *Cedrus atlantica*

♦ **Applications:** acne, dandruff, dermatitis, eczema, fungal infections, greasy skin, hair loss, skin eruptions, ulcers, arthritis, rheumatism, bronchitis, catarrh, congestion, coughs, cystitis, leucorrhoea, itches, nervous tension, and stress-related conditions

◆ **Attributes:** antiseptic, anti-putrescent, anti-seborrheic, aphrodisiac, astringent, diuretic, expectorant, fungicidal, mucolytic, sedative, stimulant, and tonic

◆ **Aroma:** warm and camphoraceous top note and tenaciously sweet, woody, and balsamic undertone

◆ **Ably blends with:** rosewood, bergamot, boronia, cypress, cassie, costus, jasmine, juniper, neroli, mimosa, labdanum, clary sage, rosemary, ylang-ylang, Oriental and floral bases

◆ **Abundant areas:** native to the Atlas Mountains of Algeria

◆ **Acquisition:** steam distillation of leaves

◆ **Areas of safety:** non-toxic, non-irritant, and non-sensitivity | do not use during pregnancy

26-CEDARWOOD (TEXAS, MEXICAN JUNIPER)

◆ **Attached Latin name:** *Juniperus ashei*
◆ **Applications:** acne, dandruff, eczema, greasy hair, insect repellent, oily skin, psoriasis, arthritis, rheumatism, bronchitis, catarrh, congestion, coughs,

sinusitis, cystitis, leucorrhoea, nervous tension, and stress-related disorders

♦ **Attributes:** antiseptic, antispasmodic, astringent, diuretic, expectorant, sedative, and stimulant

♦ **Aroma:** crude oil—smoky woody sweet tar-like odor | rectified oil—sweet, balsamic, pencil-wood

♦ **Ably blends with:** patchouli, spruce, vetiver, pine, and leather-type scents

♦ **Abundant areas:** native to Southwestern USA, Mexico, and Central America

♦ **Acquisition:** steam distillation of leaves and bark

♦ **Areas of safety:** non-toxic, but possibly an acute local irritant and may cause sensitivity | do not use during pregnancy

27-CEDARWOOD (VIRGINIA)

♦ **Attached Latin name:** *Juniperus virginiana*

♦ **Applications:** acne, dandruff, eczema, greasy hair, insect repellent, oily skin, psoriasis, arthritis, rheumatism, bronchitis, catarrh, congestion, coughs, sinusitis, cystitis, leucorrhoea, nervous tension, and stress-related disorders

♦ **Attributes:** abortifacient, anti-seborrheic, antiseptic, antispasmodic, astringent, balsamic, diuretic, emmenagogue, expectorant, insecticide, sedative, and stimulant

♦ **Aroma:** mild, sweet, balsamic, and pencil-wood

♦ **Ably blends with:** sandalwood, roses, juniper, cypress, vetiver, patchouli, and benzoin

♦ **Abundant areas:** native to North America and the Rocky Mountains

♦ **Acquisition:** steam distillation of leaves and bark

♦ **Areas of safety:** non-toxic, but possibly an acute local irritant and may cause sensitivity | do not use during pregnancy

28-CELERY

♦ **Attached Latin name:** *Apium graveolens*

♦ **Applications:** arthritis, the buildup of toxins in the blood, gout, rheumatism, dyspepsia, flatulence, indigestion, liver congestion, jaundice, amenorrhea, glandular problems, increases milk flow, cystitis, neuralgia, and sciatica

♦ **Attributes:** anti-oxidative, anti-rheumatic, antiseptic, antispasmodic, aperitif, depurative, digestive, diuretic, carminative, cholagogue, emmenagogue, galactagogic, hepatic, nervine, sedative, stimulant, stomachic, and tonic

◆ **Aroma:** spicy, warm, sweet, and long lasting

◆ **Ably blends with:** lavender, pine, lovage, oakmoss, coriander, and other spices

◆ **Abundant areas:** native to Southern Europe, cultivated as a domestic vegetable

◆ **Acquisition:** steam distillation of leaves

◆ **Areas of safety:** non-toxic and non-irritant, but may cause sensitivity | do not use during pregnancy

29-CHAMOMILE (GERMAN)

◆ **Attached Latin name:** *Matricaria chamomilla*

◆ **Applications:** acne, allergies, boils, burns, cuts, chilblains, dermatitis, earache, eczema, hair care, inflammations, insect bites, rashes, sensitive skin, teething pain, toothache, wounds, arthritis, inflamed joints, muscular pain, neuralgia, rheumatism, sprains, dyspepsia, colic, indigestion, nausea, dysmenorrhea, menopausal problems, menorrhagia, headache, insomnia, nervous tension, migraine, and stress-related conditions

◆ **Attributes:** analgesic, anti-allergenic, anti-inflammatory, antiphlogistic, antispasmodic, bactericidal, carminative, cicatrizant, cholagogue, digestive, emmenagogue, febrifuge, fungicidal, hepatic, nerve sedative, a stimulant of leucocyte production, stomachic, sudorific, vermifuge, and vulnerary

💧 **Aroma:** strong, sweet, warm, and herbaceous

💧 **Ably blends with:** geranium, lavender, patchouli, rose, benzoin, neroli, bergamot, marjoram, lemon, ylang-ylang, jasmine, clary sage, and labdanum.

💧 **Abundant areas:** native to Europe and North and West Asia, cultivated in Hungary and Eastern Europe

💧 **Acquisition:** steam distillation of leaves | absolute produced in small quantities

💧 **Areas of safety:** non-toxic and non-irritant, but may cause dermatitis in some

30-CHAMOMILE (MOROCCAN)

💧 **Attached Latin name:** *Ormenis multicaulis*

💧 **Applications:** sensitive skin, colic, colitis, headache, insomnia, irritability, migraine, amenorrhea, dysmenorrhea, menopause, and liver or spleen congestion

💧 **Attributes:** antispasmodic, cholagogue, emmenagogue, hepatic, sedative

💧 **Aroma:** fresh and herbaceous top note and a sweet, rich balsamic undertone

♦ **Ably blends with:** lavender, lavandin, cypress, cedarwood, oakmoss, and labdanum

♦ **Abundant areas:** native to Northwest Africa and Southern Spain

♦ **Acquisition:** steam distillation of leaves

♦ **Areas of safety:** non-toxic and non-irritant

31-CHAMOMILE (ROMAN)

♦ **Attached Latin name:** *Arthemis nobilis*

♦ **Applications:** sensitive skin, colic, colitis, headache, insomnia, irritability, migraine, amenorrhea, dysmenorrhea, menopause, and liver or spleen congestion

♦ **Attributes:** analgesic, anti-anemic, anti-neuralgic, antiphlogistic, antiseptic, antispasmodic, bactericidal, carminative, cholagogue, cicatrizant, digestive, emmenagogue, febrifuge, hepatic, hypnotic, nerve sedative, stomachic, sudorific, tonic, vermifuge, and vulnerary

♦ **Aroma:** warm, sweet, fruity, and herbaceous

♦ **Ably blends with:** bergamot, clary sage, oakmoss, jasmine, labdanum, neroli, rose, geranium, and lavender

♦ **Abundant areas:** native to Southern and Western Europe, cultivated in England, Belgium, Hungary, United States, Italy, and France

♦ **Acquisition:** steam distillation of leaves

♦ **Areas of safety:** non-toxic and non-irritant, but may cause dermatitis in some

32-CINNAMON

♦ **Attached Latin name:** *Cinnamomum verum*

♦ **Applications:** leaf oil only—lice, scabies, tooth and gum care, warts, wasp stings, poor circulations, rheumatism, anorexia, colitis, diarrhea, dyspepsia, intestinal infection sluggish digestion, spasm, childbirth, frigidity, leucorrhoea, metrorrhagia, scanty periods, chills, flu, infectious diseases, debility, nervous exhaustion, and stress-related conditions

♦ **Attributes:** antihelmintic, antidiarrheal, an antidote to poison, antimicrobial, antiseptic, antispasmodic, anti-putrescent, anti-parasitic, aphrodisiac, astringent, carminative, digestive, emmenagogue, hemostatic, anorexigenic, refrigerant, spasmolytic, stimulant, stomachic, and vermifuge

♦ **Aroma:** tenaciously sweet, warm, spicy, dry

♦ **Ably blends with:** ylang-ylang, orange, mandarin, benzoin, balsam of Peru, and Oriental type mixtures

♦ **Abundant areas:** native to Sri Lanka, Madagascar, Comoro Islands, South India, Burma, and Indochina, cultivated in India, Jamaica, and Africa

♦ **Acquisition:** steam distillation of leaves

♦ **Areas of safety:** leaf oil—non-toxic although possible irritant | bark oil—dermal toxin, irritant, and causes sensitivity

33-CITRONELLA

♦ **Attached Latin name:** *Cymbopogon*

♦ **Applications:** excessive perspiration, oily skin, insect repellent, colds, flu, minor infections, fatigue, headaches, migraine, and neuralgia

♦ **Attributes:** antiseptic, antispasmodic, bactericidal, deodorant, diaphoretic, diuretic, emmenagogue, febrifuge, fungicidal, insecticide, stomachic, tonic, and vermifuge

♦ **Aroma:** fresh and powerful lemony

♦ **Ably blends with:** geranium, lemon, bergamot, orange, cedarwood, and pine

♦ **Abundant areas:** native to Sri Lanka, cultivated on the southernmost tip of the country
♦ **Acquisition:** steam distillation of leaves
♦ **Areas of safety:** non-toxic and non-irritant, but may cause dermatitis in some | do not use during pregnancy

34-CORIANDER

♦ **Attached Latin name:** *Coriandrum sativum*
♦ **Applications:** accumulation of fluids or toxins, arthritis, gout, muscular aches and pains, poor circulation, rheumatism, stiffness, anorexia, colic, diarrhea, dyspepsia, flatulence, nausea, piles, spasm, colds, flu, infections, measles, debility, migraine, neuralgia, and nervous exhaustion
♦ **Attributes:** analgesic, aperitif, aphrodisiac, anti-oxidant, anti-rheumatic, antispasmodic, bactericidal, depurative, digestive, carminative, cytotoxic, fungicidal, larvicidal, lipolytic, revitalizing, stimulant, and stomachic
♦ **Aroma:** sweet, woody, spicy, and slightly musky
♦ **Ably blends with:** clary sage, bergamot, jasmine, neroli, petitgrain, citronella, sandalwood, cypress, pine, ginger, opopanax, cinnamon, and other spice oils

♦ **Abundant areas:** native to Europe and Western Asia, cultivated throughout the world, produced in the USSR, Yugoslavia, and Romania

♦ **Acquisition:** steam distillation of leaves

♦ **Areas of safety:** non-toxic

35-CLOVE

♦ **Attached Latin name:** *Syzygium aromaticum*

♦ **Applications:** asthma, bronchitis, rheumatism, exhaustion, infection, burns, cuts, arthritis, diarrhea, colds, and hernia; also used as a mosquito repellent, and in perfume, liqueurs, mulled wine, dental products, and love potions

♦ **Attributes:** lowest percentage of the chemical component eugenol | antiseptic, antiviral, antibiotic, stimulant, expectorant, and aphrodisiac

♦ **Aroma:** powerfully sweet, spicy, fruity, and warm

♦ **Ably blends with:** roses, orange, bergamot, cinnamon, cloves, caraway, ylang-ylang, labdanum, cedarwood, neroli, and Oriental bases

♦ **Abundant areas:** native to Indonesia and Madagascar, cultivated in the Philippines and Molucca Islands

♦ **Acquisition:** steam distillation of dried flower buds, leaves, and stems

♦ **Areas of safety:** handled with caution as it easily irritates the skin

36-COSTUS

♦ **Attached Latin name:** *Chamaecostus cuspidatus*

♦ **Applications:** perfume, asthma, bronchitis, spasmodic cough, flatulence, indigestion, spasm, debility, nervous exhaustion, and other stress-related conditions

♦ **Attributes:** antiseptic, antispasmodic, antiviral, bactericidal, carminative, digestive, expectorant, febrifuge, hypotensive, stimulant, stomachic, and tonic

♦ **Aroma:** tenaciously woody and musty

♦ **Ably blends with:** patchouli, ylang-ylang, floral, and Oriental fragrances

♦ **Abundant areas:** native to Northern India, cultivated in India and Southwest China

♦ **Acquisition:** steam distillation of macerated dried roots followed by solvent extraction with distilled water

♦ **Areas of safety:** non-toxic and non-irritant, but may cause sensitivity in some

37-Cubeb

♦ **Attached Latin name:** *Piper cubeba*
♦ **Applications:** bronchitis, catarrh, congestion, chronic coughs, sinusitis, throat infections, flatulence, indigestion, perfumery, sluggish digestion, cystitis, leucorrhea, and urethritis
♦ **Attributes:** antiseptic, antispasmodic, antiviral, bactericidal, carminative, diuretic, expectorant, and stimulant
♦ **Aroma:** warm, woody, spicy, and slightly camphoraceous
♦ **Ably blends with:** ylang-ylang, galbanum, lavender, rosemary, black pepper, allspice, and other spices
♦ **Abundant areas:** native to Indonesia, cultivated throughout Southeast Africa
♦ **Acquisition:** steam distillation of leaves
♦ **Areas of safety:** non-toxic, non-irritant, and non-sensitivity

38-CUMIN

♦ **Attached Latin name:** *Cuminum cyminum*

♦ **Applications:** accumulation of fluids or toxins, poor circulation, colic, dyspepsia, flatulence, indigestion, spasm, debility, headaches, migraine, and nervous exhaustion

♦ **Attributes:** anti-oxidant, antiseptic, antispasmodic, antitoxic, aphrodisiac, bactericidal, carminative, depurative, digestive, diuretic, emmenagogue, larvicidal, nervine, stimulant, and tonic

♦ **Aroma:** warm, soft, spicy, and musky

♦ **Ably blends with:** lavender, lavandin, rosemary, galbanum, rosewood, cardamom, and Oriental-type fragrances

♦ **Abundant areas:** native to Northern Egypt, cultivated in the Mediterranean, Spain, France, and Morocco

♦ **Acquisition:** steam distillation of leaves

♦ **Areas of safety:** non-toxic, non-irritant, and non-sensitivity | do not use during pregnancy | do not expose treated skin to direct sunlight

39-CYPRESS

- **Attached Latin name:** *Cupressus*
- **Applications:** hemorrhoids, oily and overhydrated skin, excessive perspiration, insect repellent, pyorrhea, varicose veins, wounds, cellulitis, muscular cramp, edema, poor circulations, rheumatism, asthma, bronchitis, spasmodic coughing, dysmenorrhea, menopausal problems, menorrhagia, nervous tension, and stress-related conditions
- **Attributes:** anti-rheumatic, antiseptic, antispasmodic, astringent, deodorant, diuretic, hepatic, styptic, sudorific, tonic, and vasoconstrictive

- **Aroma:** tenaciously smoky, sweet, and balsamic
- **Ably blends with:** cedarwood, pine, lavender, mandarin, clary sage, lemon, cardamom, Moroccan chamomile, ambrette seed, labdanum, juniper, benzoin, bergamot, orange, marjoram, and sandalwood
- **Abundant areas:** native to the Eastern Mediterranean region, grows wild in France, Italy, Corsica, Sardinia, Sicily, Spain, Portugal, North Africa, England, and the Balkan countries
- **Acquisition:** steam distillation of needles and twigs with occasional oil productions from cones

◊ **Areas of safety:** non-toxic, non-irritant, and non-sensitivity

40-DILL

◊ **Attached Latin name:** *Anethum graveolens*
◊ **Applications:** dyspepsia, lack of periods, colic, flatulence, and indigestion
◊ **Attributes:** antispasmodic, bactericidal, carminative, digestive, emmenagogue, galactagogic, hypotensive, stimulant, and stomachic
◊ **Aroma:** powerfully sweet, and spicy
◊ **Ably blends with:** elemi, spice, nutmeg, and citrus oils
◊ **Abundant areas:** native to the Mediterranean and the Black Sea regions, cultivated worldwide
◊ **Acquisition:** steam distillation of leaves
◊ **Areas of safety:** non-toxic, non-irritant, and non-sensitivity

41-ELEMI

◊ **Attached Latin name:** *Canarium luzonicum*
◊ **Applications:** bronchitis, catarrhal conditions, unproductive coughs, aged skin, infected cuts and

wounds, inflammations, wrinkles, nervous exhaustion, and stress-related conditions

♦ **Attributes:** antiseptic, balsamic, cicatrizant, expectorant, fortifying, regulatory, stimulant, stomachic, and tonic

♦ **Aroma:** light, fresh, balsamic, spicy, lemon-like

♦ **Ably blends with:** cinnamon, sage, lavandin, lavender, rosemary, labdanum, frankincense, myrrh, and other spices

♦ **Abundant areas:** native to the Philippine Islands and the Moluccas

♦ **Acquisition:** steam distillation of leaves

♦ **Areas of safety:** non-toxic, non-irritant, and non-sensitivity

42-EUCALYPTUS

♦ **Attached Latin name:** *Eucalyptus globulus*

♦ **Applications:** asthma, bronchitis, catarrh, coughs, throat and mouth infections, headaches, nervous exhaustion, neuralgia, sciatica, cuts, sores, ulcers, colds, fevers, flu, infectious illnesses (measles), arthritis, muscular aches/pains, rheumatism, sports injuries, and sprains

♦ **Attributes:** analgesic, anti-neuralgic, anti-parasitic, anti-rheumatic, antiseptic, antispasmodic, antiviral, balsamic, cicatrizant, decongestant, deodorant, depurative, diuretic, expectorant, febrifuge, hypoglycemic, prophylactic, rubefacient, stimulant, vermifuge, and vulnerary

♦ **Aroma:** fresh, camphoraceous, spicy, and minty

♦ **Ably blends with:** lemon, cedarwood, pine, marjoram, lavender, and rosemary

♦ **Abundant areas:** native to Tasmania and Australia

♦ **Acquisition:** steam distillation of leaves

♦ **Areas of safety:** non-toxic, non-irritant, and non-sensitivity

43-EUCALYPTUS (BLUE GUM)

♦ **Attached Latin name:** *Eucalyptus globulus Labill*

♦ **Applications:** debility, headaches, neuralgia, burns, blisters, cuts, herpes, insect bites, insect repellent, lice, skin infections, wounds, chickenpox, colds, epidemics, measles, muscular aches and pains, poor circulation, rheumatoid arthritis, sprains, cystitis, leucorrhoea, asthma, bronchitis, catarrh, coughs, sinusitis, and throat infections

◆ **Attributes:** analgesic, anti-neuralgic, anti-parasitic, anti-rheumatic, antiseptic, antispasmodic, antiviral, balsamic, cicatrizant, decongestant, deodorant, depurative, diuretic, expectorant, febrifuge, hypoglycemic, prophylactic, rubefacient, stimulant, vermifuge, and vulnerary

◆ **Aroma:** harshly camphoraceous with a woody and sweet undertone

◆ **Ably blends with:** lemon, cedarwood, pine, marjoram, lavender, and rosemary

◆ **Abundant areas:** native to Tasmania and Australia, cultivated in Spain, Portugal, Brazil, California, Russia, and China

◆ **Acquisition:** steam distillation of leaves

◆ **Areas of safety:** non-toxic, non-irritant, and non-sensitivity

44-EUCALYPTUS (LEMON-SCENTED)

◆ **Attached Latin name:** *Corymbia citriodora*

◆ **Applications:** colds, fevers, infectious skin conditions (chickenpox), Athlete's foot, cuts, dandruff, herpes, insect repellent, scabs, sores, wounds, asthma, laryngitis, and sore throat

◆ **Attributes:** antiseptic, antiviral, bactericidal, deodorant, expectorant, fungicidal, and insecticide

◆ **Aroma:** strong, sweet, fresh, citronella-like, and balsamic undertone

◆ **Ably blends with:** cedarwood, pine, marjoram, lavender, and rosemary

◆ **Abundant areas:** native to Australia, cultivated in Brazil and China

◆ **Acquisition:** steam distillation of leaves

◆ **Areas of safety:** non-toxic, non-irritant, and non-sensitivity

45-FENNEL (SWEET)

◆ **Attached Latin name:** *Foeniculum vulgare*

◆ **Applications:** sweet fennel only—bruises, dull oily mature complexions, pyorrhea, amenorrhea, insufficient milk in nursing mothers, menopausal problems, cellulitis, obesity, edema, rheumatism, anorexia, colic, constipation, dyspepsia, flatulence, hiccough, nausea, asthma, and bronchitis

◆ **Attributes:** aperitif, anti-inflammatory, antimicrobial, antiseptic, antispasmodic, carminative, depurative, diuretic, emmenagogue, expectorant, galactagogic, laxative, anorexigenic, stimulant, splenic, stomachic, tonic, and vermifuge

♦ **Aroma:** sweet anise-like, slightly earthy, and peppery scent | seed oil sharp, warm, and camphoraceous

♦ **Ably blends with:** geranium, lavender, roses, and sandalwood

♦ **Abundant areas:** native to Malta, cultivated in France, Italy, and Greece

♦ **Acquisition:** steam distillation of leaves

♦ **Areas of safety:** non-toxic and non-irritant, but may cause sensitivity in some | narcotic in large doses

46-FIR NEEDLE

♦ **Attached Latin name:** *Abies alba*

♦ **Applications:** colds, fever, flu, arthritis, muscular aches/pains, rheumatism, bronchitis, coughs, and sinusitis

♦ **Attributes:** analgesic, antiseptic, antitussive, deodorant, expectorant, rubefacient, stimulant, and tonic

♦ **Aroma:** pleasing, rich, sweet, and balsamic

🜕 **Ably blends with:** galbanum, labdanum, lavender, rosemary, lemon, pine, and marjoram

🜕 **Abundant areas:** native to mountainous regions of Northern Europe, cultivated in Switzerland, Poland, Germany, France, Austria, and Yugoslavia

🜕 **Acquisition:** steam distillation of leaves

🜕 **Areas of safety:** non-toxic, non-irritant, and non-sensitivity

47-FRANKINCENSE

🜕 **Attached Latin name:** *Boswellia*

🜕 **Applications:** cystitis, dysmenorrhea, leucorrhoea, metrorrhagia, blemishes, dry/mature complexions, scars, wounds, wrinkles, anxiety, nervous tension/stress related conditions, asthma, bronchitis, catarrh, coughs, and laryngitis

🜕 **Attributes:** anti-inflammatory, antiseptic, astringent, carminative, cicatrizant, cytophylactic, digestive, diuretic, emmenagogue, expectorant, sedative, tonic, uterine, and vulnerary

🜕 **Aroma:** fresh top note with a warm, rich, sweet, and balsamic undertone

● **Ably blends with:** cinnamon, pepper, basil, camphor, bergamot, orange, opopanax, neroli, mimosa, lavender, geranium, pine, sandalwood, and other spices

● **Abundant areas:** native to the Red Sea region, grows wild throughout Northeast Africa

● **Acquisition:** steam distillation of leaves

● **Areas of safety:** non-toxic, non-irritant, and non-sensitivity

48-GALANGAL

● **Attached Latin name:** *Alpinia galanga*

● **Applications:** possibly digestive

● **Attributes:** antiseptic, bactericidal, carminative, diaphoretic, stimulant, and stomachic

● **Aroma:** fresh, spicy, and camphoraceous

● **Ably blends with:** Moroccan chamomile, sage, cinnamon, allspice, lavandin, pine needle, rosemary, patchouli, opopanax, and citrus oils

● **Abundant areas:** native to Southeast China, cultivated in Indonesia, Thailand, and Japan

● **Acquisition:** steam distillation of the leaves

● **Areas of safety:** no data available

49-GALBANUM

- **Attached Latin name:** *Ferula galbanifua*
- **Applications:** nervous tension/stress related complaints, abscesses, acne, boils, cuts, scar tissue, inflammations, tones, wrinkles, wounds, cramp, flatulence, indigestion, muscular aches/pains, poor circulation, rheumatism, asthma, bronchitis, catarrh, and chronic coughs
- **Attributes:** analgesic, anti-inflammatory, antimicrobial, antiseptic, antispasmodic, aphrodisiac, balsamic, carminative, cicatrizant, digestive, diuretic, emmenagogue, expectorant, hypotensive, restorative, and tonic
- **Aroma:** fresh green top note with a woody, dry, and balsamic undertone
- **Ably blends with:** hyacinth, lavender, geranium oakmoss, pine, fir, and Oriental bases
- **Abundant areas:** native to the Middle East and Western Asia, cultivated Iran, Turkey, Afghanistan, and Lebanon
- **Acquisition:** steam distillation of leaves
- **Areas of safety:** non-toxic, non-irritant, and non-sensitivity

50-Gardenia

- **Attached Latin name:** *Gardenia jasminoides*
- **Applications:** perfume
- **Attributes:** antiseptic and aphrodisiac
- **Aroma:** sweet, rich, floral, and jasmine-like
- **Ably blends with:** ylang-ylang, jasmine, neroli, rose, spice, and citrus oils
- **Abundant areas:** native to the Far East, India, and China
- **Acquisition:** absolute—solvent extraction
- **Areas of safety:** no data available

51-Garlic

- **Attached Latin name:** *Allium sativum*
- **Applications:** not used externally due to smell | taken internally through capsules for respiratory/gastrointestinal infections etc.
- **Attributes:** amebicidal, antihelmintic, antibiotic, anti-hypocholesterolemia, antimicrobial, antiseptic, antitoxic, anti-tumor, antiviral, bactericidal, carminative, cholagogue, depurative, diaphoretic, diuretic, expectorant, febrifuge, fungicidal,

hypoglycemic, hypotensive, insecticidal, larvicidal, promotes leukocytosis, stomachic, and tonic

- **Aroma:** strong and unpleasant
- **Ably blends with:** no data available
- **Abundant areas:** native to Southwest Siberia and spread to Europe and central Asia
- **Acquisition:** steam distillation of leaves
- **Areas of safety:** non-toxic and non-irritant, but may irritate the stomach and cause sensitivity in some

52-GERANIUM

- **Attached Latin name:** *Pelargonium*
- **Applications:** nervous tension, neuralgia, stress-related conditions, acne, bruises, broken capillaries, burns, congested skin, mature skin, cuts, dermatitis, eczema, , ulcers, hemorrhoids, lice, mosquito repellent, oily complexion, wounds, menopausal problems, cellulitis, adrenocortical glands, engorgement of breasts, edema, ringworm, and poor circulation
- **Attributes:** antidepressant, anti-hemorrhagic, anti-inflammatory, antiseptic, astringent, cicatrizant, deodorant, diuretic, fungicidal, hemostatic, stimulant, styptic, tonic, vermifuge, and vulnerary
- **Aroma:** green, rosy, sweet, and minty

⚫ **Ably blends with:** lavender, patchouli, clove, roses, sandalwood, jasmine, juniper, neroli, bergamot, and citrus oils

⚫ **Abundant areas:** native to South Africa, cultivated in Japan, Russia, Congo, Egypt, Central America, and Europe

⚫ **Acquisition:** steam distillation of leaves

⚫ **Areas of safety:** non-toxic, non-irritant, and non-sensitivity, but may cause contact dermatitis

53-GINGER

⚫ **Attached Latin name:** *Zingiber officinale*

⚫ **Applications:** arthritis, fatigue, muscular aches/pains, strains, sprains, rheumatism, poor circulation, catarrh, congestion, coughs, sinusitis, sore throat, diarrhea, colic, cramp, flatulence, indigestion, loss of appetite, nausea, travel sickness, CHILD syndrome, colds, fever, flu, debility, infectious disease, and nervous exhaustion

⚫ **Attributes:** analgesic, aphrodisiac, aperitif, anti-oxidant, antitussive, antiseptic, antispasmodic, bactericidal, carminative, cephalic, diaphoretic, expectorant, stomachic, stimulant, febrifuge, rubefacient, laxative, and tonic

♦ **Aroma:** warm, slightly green, fresh, woody, and spicy

♦ **Ably blends with:** coriander, roses, lime, neroli, orange, sandalwood, vetiver, patchouli, and citrus oils

♦ **Abundant areas:** native to Southern Asia, cultivated in the tropics, Nigeria, West Indies, India, China, Jamaica, and Japan

♦ **Acquisition:** steam distillation of leaves

♦ **Areas of safety:** non-toxic, non-irritant, but slightly phototoxic and may cause sensitivity

54-GRAPEFRUIT

♦ **Attached Latin name:** *Citrus paradisi*

♦ **Applications:** cellulitis, exercise preparation, muscle nervous exhaustion, fatigue, headaches, obesity, colds, stiffness, chills, depression, water retention, performance stress, acne, congested/oily skin, promotes hair growth, and tones skin, and tissues

♦ **Attributes:** antiseptic, antitoxic, astringent, bactericidal, diuretic, depurative, stimulant and tonic

♦ **Aroma:** fresh, sweet, and citrus

♦ **Ably blends with:** lavender, geranium, lemon, palmarosa, bergamot, neroli, rosemary, cardamom, and spice oils

◆ **Abundant areas:** native to tropical Asia and the West Indies, cultivated in Brazil, Florida, California, and Israel

◆ **Acquisition:** steam distillation of berries

◆ **Areas of safety:** non-toxic, non-irritant, but slightly phototoxic and may cause sensitivity

55-GUAIAC WOOD

◆ **Attached Latin name:** *Guaiacum officinale*

◆ **Applications:** arthritis, gout, and rheumatoid arthritis

◆ **Attributes:** anti-inflammatory, antioxidant, anti-rheumatic, antiseptic, diaphoretic, diuretic, and laxative

◆ **Aroma:** pleasant, tea rose-type fragrance, sometimes with smoky undertones

◆ **Ably blends with:** spice, geranium, amyris, neroli, sandalwood, oakmoss, costus, and roses

◆ **Abundant areas:** native to Paraguay and Argentina

◆ **Acquisition:** steam distillation of leaves

◆ **Areas of safety:** non-toxic, non-irritant, and non-sensitivity

56-HELICHRYSUM (EVERLASTING | IMMORTELLE)

♦ **Attached Latin name:** *Helichrysum orientale*

♦ **Applications:** depression, debility, lethargy, nervous exhaustion, neuralgia, stress-related conditions, abscess, flu, acne, colds, allergic conditions, eczema, bacterial infections, boils, wounds, burns, spots, cuts, inflammation, dermatitis, fever, muscular aches/pains, rheumatism, sprains, strained muscles, liver / spleen congestion, asthma, bronchitis, and chronic whooping coughs

♦ **Attributes:** anti-allergenic, anti-inflammatory, antimicrobial, antitussive, antiseptic, astringent, cholagogue, cicatrizant, diuretic, expectorant, fungicidal, hepatic, and nervine

♦ **Aroma:** powerful, rich, and honey-like with a delicate, tea-like undertone

♦ **Ably blends with:** chamomile, clove, boronia, balsam of Peru, labdanum, roses, lavender, clary sage, mimosa, oakmoss, and geranium

♦ **Abundant areas:** native to the Mediterranean areas, cultivated in Spain, Yugoslavia, Italy, and France

♦ **Acquisition:** oil—a steam distillation of leaves | absolute—solvent extraction

♦ **Areas of safety:** non-toxic, non-irritant, and non-sensitivity

57-HOPS

♦ **Attached Latin name:** *Humulus lupulus*
♦ **Applications:** headaches, insomnia, nervous tension, neuralgia, stress-related conditions, rough skin, rashes, dermatitis, ulcers, amenorrhea, menstrual cramp, supports female estrogens, promotes feminine characteristics, reduces sexual overactivity, asthma, spasmodic cough, indigestion, and nervous dyspepsia
♦ **Attributes:** anodyne, aphrodisiac, antiseptic, antispasmodic, astringent, bactericidal, carminative, diuretic, emollient, estrogenic properties, hypnotic, nervine, sedative, and soporific
♦ **Aroma:** rich, spicy, and sweet
♦ **Ably blends with:** nutmeg, pine, citrus, hyacinth, copaiba balsam, and spice oils.
♦ **Abundant areas:** native to North America and Europe, cultivated worldwide
♦ **Acquisition:** oil—a steam distillation of leaves | absolute—solvent extraction
♦ **Areas of safety:** non-toxic and nonirritant, but may cause *sensitivity* in some

58-HYACINTH

♦ **Attached Latin name:** *Hyacinthus*
♦ **Applications:** described as *'refreshing and invigorating to a tired mind'* | also used for stress-related conditions
♦ **Attributes:** antiseptic, balsamic, hypnotic, sedative, and styptic
♦ **Aroma:** sweet, green, and floral with a soft floral undertone
♦ **Ably blends with:** neroli, violet, jasmine, ylang-ylang, and galbanum
♦ **Abundant areas:** native to Asia Minor, cultivated mainly in Holland and Southern France
♦ **Acquisition:** solvent extraction of concrete and absolute
♦ **Areas of safety:** no data available

59-HYSSOP

♦ **Attached Latin name:** *Hyssopus officinalis*
♦ **Applications:** anxiety, fatigue, nervous tension, rheumatism, bruises, low/high blood pressure, flu, colds, dermatitis, cuts, inflammation, eczema, wounds,

amenorrhea, leucorrhoea, asthma, bronchitis, catarrh, colic, cough, tonsillitis, sore throat, indigestion.

💧 **Attributes:** astringent, antiseptic, antispasmodic, antiviral, bactericidal, carminative, cephalic, cicatrizant, digestive, diuretic, emmenagogue, expectorant, febrifuge, hypertensive, nervine, sedative, sudorific, tonic, vermifuge, and vulnerary

💧 **Aroma:** sweet, camphoraceous top note with a warm, spicy, and herbaceous undertone

💧 **Ably blends with:** citrus oils, rosemary, geranium, bay leaf, clary sage, and lavender

💧 **Abundant areas:** native to the Mediterranean region, grows wild throughout Europe, Russia, and America, cultivated in Hungary and France

💧 **Acquisition:** steam distillation of leaves

💧 **Areas of safety:** non-irritant and non-sensitivity, but moderately toxic | do not use during pregnancy | use in moderation

60-JASMINE

💧 **Attached Latin name:** *Jasminum*

💧 **Applications:** dry, greasy, irritated, and sensitive skin, muscular spasm, sprains, catarrh, coughs, hoarseness, laryngitis, dysmenorrhea, frigidity, labor pains, uterine disorders, depression, nervous exhaustion, and stress-related conditions

⚬ **Attributes:** Mild analgesic, anti-inflammatory, antidepressant, antispasmodic, antiseptic, aphrodisiac, carminative, cicatrizant, expectorant, galactagogic, parturient, sedative, and tonic

⚬ **Aroma:** rich, warm, and floral with a tea-like undertone

⚬ **Ably blends with:** citrus oils, clary sage, roses, and sandalwood

⚬ **Abundant areas:** native to China, Northern India, and West Asia, cultivated in the Mediterranean region, China, and India

⚬ **Acquisition:** concrete—solvent extraction | absolute— alcohol separation of concrete

⚬ **Areas of safety:** non-toxic, non-irritant, and non-sensitivity

61-JUNIPER BERRY

⚬ **Attached Latin name:** *Juniperus*
⚬ **Applications:** anxiety, depression, nervous tension, stress-related conditions, amenorrhea, cystitis, leucorrhea, dysmenorrhea, dermatitis, flu, colds, infections, accumulation of toxins, acne,

arteriosclerosis, gout, cellulitis, rheumatism, obesity, eczema, hair loss, hemorrhoids, oily complexions.

💧 **Attributes:** Anti-parasitic, anti-rheumatic, antiseptic, antitoxic, antispasmodic, aphrodisiac, astringent, rubefacient, carminative, depurative, cicatrizant, diuretic, nervine, emmenagogue, sedative, stomachic, tonic, sudorific, and vulnerary

💧 **Aroma:** sweet, fresh, woody, and balsamic

💧 **Ably blends with:** vetiver, sandalwood, cedarwood, mastic, geranium, oakmoss, balsam tolu, galbanum, benzoin, elemi, rosemary, cypress, fir needle, labdanum, clary sage, lavandin, lavender, pine, and citrus oils

💧 **Abundant areas:** native to the Northern Hemisphere, Scandinavia, Siberia, Canada, Northern Europe, and Northern Asia

💧 **Acquisition:** steam distillation of berries

💧 **Areas of safety:** non-toxic and non-sensitivity, but may be slightly irritating | do not use during pregnancy

62-LABDANUM

💧 **Attached Latin name:** *Cistus ladanifer*

◆ **Applications:** mature skin, rhinitis, bronchitis, coughs, wrinkles, and colds

◆ **Attributes:** antimicrobial, antiseptic, antitussive, astringent, balsamic, emmenagogue, expectorant, and tonic

◆ **Aroma:** warm, sweet, dry, herbaceous, and musky

◆ **Ably blends with:** Moroccan chamomile, patchouli, sandalwood, vetiver, cypress, bergamot, lavandin, lavender, juniper, pine, clary sage, and oakmoss

◆ **Abundant areas:** native to the Mediterranean mountainous regions and the Middle East

◆ **Acquisition:** resin, concrete, and absolute—solvent extraction | oil—steam distillation

◆ **Areas of safety:** non-toxic, non-irritant, and non-sensitivity | do not use during pregnancy

63-LAVANDIN

◆ **Attached Latin name:** *Lavandula*

◆ **Applications:** similar to true lavender, but more rubefacient and penetrating | antispasmodic, antichlorotic, anti-parasitic, antitoxic, cholagogue, cicatrizant, carminative, cordial, cytophylactic, diuretic, deodorant, hypotensive, emmenagogue, insecticide, sedative, nervine, stimulant, sudorific, tonic, vermifuge, and vulnerary

● **Attributes:** analgesic, anticonvulsive, antidepressant, antimicrobial, anti-rheumatic, and antiseptic

● **Aroma:** fresh, camphoraceous top note with a woody and herbaceous undertone

● **Ably blends with:** clove, citronella, bay leaf, cypress, cinnamon, clary sage, pine, rosemary, geranium, patchouli, and citrus oils

● **Abundant areas:** native to the mountainous regions of Southern France, cultivated in Spain, Yugoslavia, Hungary, and Argentina

● **Acquisition:** absolute and concrete— solvent extraction | oil—steam distillation

● **Areas of safety:** non-toxic, non-irritant, and non-sensitivity

64-LAVENDER

● **Attached Latin name:** *Lavandula angustifolia*

● **Applications:** suitable for all skin types with abscesses, allergies, acne, athlete's foot, bruises, boils, burns, dermatitis, dandruff, earache, inflammations, eczema, insect bites and stings, lice, insect repellent, psoriasis, sunburn, scabies, spots, sores, ringworm, and wounds

used also for hypertension, depression, insomnia, headache, migraine, stress-related conditions, nervous tension, PMT, shock, sciatica, vertigo, muscular aches/pains, lumbago, rheumatism, sprains, flu, cystitis, dysmenorrhea, leucorrhoea, asthma, abdominal cramps, bronchitis, whooping cough, catarrh, throat infections, laryngitis, halitosis, dyspepsia, colic, flatulence, and nausea

♦ **Attributes:** analgesic, antichlorotic, antidepressant, antimicrobial, anticonvulsive, antiparasitic, anti-rheumatic, antiseptic, antispasmodic, antitoxic, cholagogue, cicatrizant, carminative, cytophylactic, diuretic, nervine, deodorant, insecticide, hypotensive, emmenagogue, rubefacient, stimulant, sedative, vermifuge, tonic, sudorific, and vulnerary

♦ **Aroma:** fresh, herbaceous, and camphoraceous

♦ **Ably blends with:** rosemary, sage, lavandin, eucalyptus, rosewood, lavender, petitgrain, pine, cedarwood, oakmoss, opopanax, patchouli, and spice oils

♦ **Abundant areas:** native to the mountainous regions of France, Spain, and North Africa, cultivated worldwide

♦ **Acquisition:** steam distillation of leaves

♦ **Areas of safety:** non-toxic, non-irritant, and non-sensitivity

65-LEMON

♦ **Attached Latin name:** *Citrus limon*

♦ **Applications:** colds, flu, dyspepsia, fever, infections, asthma, bronchitis, arthritis, catarrh, cellulitis, throat infections, high blood pressure, obesity, nosebleeds, poor circulation, acne, anemia, brittle nails, rheumatism, boils, chilblains, corns, greasy skin, cuts, herpes, insect bites, spots, mouth ulcers, varicose veins, and warts

♦ **Attributes:** anti-anemic, antimicrobial, antichlorotic, antiscorbutic, anti-rheumatic, antiseptic, antispasmodic, astringent, bactericidal, antitoxic, carminative, cicatrizant, depurative, diaphoretic, febrifuge, diuretic, hemostatic, hypotensive, insecticidal, rubefacient, stimulates white corpuscles, tonic, and vermifuge

♦ **Aroma:** light, fresh, and citrus

♦ **Ably blends with:** lavender, neroli, ylang-ylang, sandalwood, rose, chamomile, fennel, benzoin, geranium, juniper, eucalyptus, oakmoss, elemi, lavandin, and labdanum

♦ **Abundant areas:** native to Asia, grows wild in the Mediterranean, cultivated extensively worldwide in Italy, Sicily, Cyprus, South and North America, Israel, and Guinea

♦ **Acquisition:** cold press expression

♦ **Areas of safety:** non-toxic, but may cause dermal irritation or sensitivity in some

66-LEMONGRASS

♦ **Attached Latin name:** *Cymbopogon*

♦ **Applications:** acne, athlete's foot, excessive perspiration, open pores, insect repellent, pediculosis, tissue toner, scabies, fevers, headaches, infectious disease, gastroenteritis, stress-related conditions, nervous exhaustion, colitis, indigestion, muscular pain, muscle tone/poor circulation, and slack tissue

♦ **Attributes:** analgesic, antidepressant, antimicrobial, anti-oxidant, antipyretic, antiseptic, bactericidal, astringent, deodorant, carminative, febrifuge, fungicidal, galactagogic, insecticidal, nervine, sedative, and tonic

◆ **Aroma:** fresh, grassy, and citrus with an earthy undertone

◆ **Ably blends with:** no data available

◆ **Abundant areas:** native to Asia, and Sri Lanka, cultivated in West and East India

◆ **Acquisition:** steam distillation of leaves

◆ **Areas of safety:** non-toxic, but a possible dermal irritant and may cause sensitivity in some

67-LIME

◆ **Attached Latin name:** *Citrus aurantiifolia*

◆ **Applications:** colds, fever, flu, dyspepsia, infections, throat infections, asthma, bronchitis, catarrh, cellulitis, nosebleeds, arthritis, greasy skin, high blood pressure, rheumatism, obesity, chilblains, poor circulation, brittle nails, acne, anemia, herpes, corns, boils, cuts, mouth ulcers, spots, insect bites, varicose veins, and warts

◆ **Attributes:** anti-rheumatic, antiscorbutic, antiseptic, antiviral, aperitif, bactericidal, febrifuge, restorative, and tonic

◆ **Aroma:** fresh, sharp, fruity, and citrus

- **Ably blends with:** clary sage, rosemary, lavandin, lavender, citronella, and neroli
- **Abundant areas:** native to South Asia, cultivated in South Florida, Central America, the West Indies, and Italy
- **Acquisition:** cold press expression of peel, or steam distillation of the completely ripe, crushed fruit
- **Areas of safety:** non-toxic, non-irritant, and non-sensitivity

68-LINALOE

- **Attached Latin name:** *Bursera delpechiana*
- **Applications:** acne, cuts, wounds, dermatitis, nervous tension, and stress-related conditions
- **Attributes:** anticonvulsant, anti-inflammatory, antiseptic, bactericidal, deodorant, and gentle tonic
- **Aroma:** sweet, woody, and floral
- **Ably blends with:** roses, cedarwood, rosewood, sandalwood, frankincense, woody, and floral fragrances
- **Abundant areas:** native to South and Central America, cultivated in the Far East
- **Acquisition:** steam distillation of leaves
- **Areas of safety:** non-toxic, non-irritant, and non-sensitivity

69-LOVAGE

- **Attached Latin name:** *Levisticum officinale*
- **Applications:** amenorrhea, dysmenorrhea, cystitis, flatulence, anemia, spasm, indigestion, congestion, accumulation of toxins, gout, edema, poor circulation, rheumatism, and water retention
- **Attributes:** antimicrobial, antiseptic, antispasmodic, digestive, diaphoretic, diuretic, depurative, carminative, emmenagogue, febrifuge, expectorant, stimulant, and stomachic
- **Aroma:** rich, spicy, warm, and root-like
- **Ably blends with:** roses, galbanum, costus, bay, oakmoss, lavandin, and spice oils
- **Abundant areas:** native to southern Europe and Western Asia, naturalized in North America, cultivated in Central and Southern Europe
- **Acquisition:** steam distillation of the fresh roots and the herb
- **Areas of safety:** non-toxic, non-irritant, and non-sensitivity

70-MANDARIN (TANGERINE)

◊ **Attached Latin name:** *Citrus tangerina*
◊ **Applications:** acne, congestion, oily skin, spots, scars, stretch marks, insomnia, toner, nervous tension, fluid retention, restlessness, obesity, dyspepsia, digestive problems, hiccoughs, and intestinal problems
◊ **Attributes:** antiseptic, antispasmodic, carminative, digestive, diuretic, laxative, sedative, stimulant, and tonic
◊ **Aroma:** intensely sweet, almost floral, and citrus
◊ **Ably blends with:** other citrus oils, neroli, clove, cinnamon, nutmeg, and other spice oils
◊ **Abundant areas:** native to the Far East and Southern China, cultivated in Italy, Spain, Algeria, Cyprus, the Middle East, and Brazil
◊ **Acquisition:** cold press expression of the rind
◊ **Areas of safety:** non-toxic, non-irritant, and non-sensitivity, possibly phototoxic

71-MARIGOLD

◊ **Attached Latin name:** *Tagetes*
◊ **Applications:** burns, cuts, eczema, greasy skin, inflammations, insect bites, rashes, and wounds

🜄 **Attributes:** anti-hemorrhagic, anti-inflammatory, antiseptic, antispasmodic, astringent, diaphoretic, cholagogue, cicatrizant, emmenagogue, febrifuge, fungicidal, styptic, tonic, and vulnerary

🜄 **Aroma:** intensely sharp, and herbaceous

🜄 **Ably blends with:** oakmoss, hyacinth, and citrus oils

🜄 **Abundant areas:** native to southern Europe and Egypt, cultivated in northern Europe; France only produces the absolute

🜄 **Acquisition:** absolute—solvent extraction of the flowers

🜄 **Areas of safety:** non-toxic, non-irritant, and non-sensitivity

72-MARJORAM

🜄 **Attached Latin name:** *Origanum majorana*

🜄 **Applications:** chilblains, bruises, ticks, headache, hypertension, insomnia, migraine, nervous tension and stress-related conditions, arthritis, lumbago, muscular aches/stiffness, rheumatism, sprains, strains, colds, asthma, bronchitis, coughs, amenorrhea, dysmenorrhea, leucorrhoea AMP, colic, constipation, dyspepsia, and flatulence

◆ **Attributes:** analgesic, aphrodisiac, anti-oxidant, antiseptic, antispasmodic, antiviral, bactericidal, carminative, cordial, diaphoretic, digestive, diuretic, emmenagogue, expectorant, fungicidal, hypotensive, laxative, nervine, sedative, stomachic, tonic, vasodilatory, and vulnerary

◆ **Aroma:** warm, woody, spicy, and camphoraceous

◆ **Ably blends with:** lavender, rosemary, bergamot, chamomile, cypress, cedarwood, and eucalyptus

◆ **Abundant areas:** native to the Mediterranean region, Egypt, and North Africa, produced by France, Tunisia, Morocco, Egypt, Bulgaria, Hungary, and Germany

◆ **Acquisition:** absolute—solvent extraction of the flowers

◆ **Areas of safety:** non-toxic, non-irritant, and non-sensitivity

73-MASTIC

◆ **Attached Latin name:** *Pistacia lentiscus*

◆ **Applications:** boils, cuts, fleas, insect repellent, lice, ringworm, scabies, wounds, neuralgia, colds, arthritis, gout, muscular aches / rheumatism, sciatica, bronchitis, catarrh, whooping cough, cystitis, leucorrhoea, and urethritis

♦ **Attributes:** antimicrobial, antiseptic, antispasmodic, astringent, diuretic, expectorant, and stimulant

♦ **Aroma:** faint, balsamic, and turpentine-like

♦ **Ably blends with:** lavender, mimosa, citrus, and floral oils

♦ **Abundant areas:** native to the Mediterranean region and North Africa, produced in the Greek Island of Chios, Algeria, Morocco, and the Canary Islands

♦ **Acquisition:** resin—solvent extraction of the oleoresin | oil—a steam distillation of the oleoresin, or occasionally, of the leaves and branches

♦ **Areas of safety:** non-toxic, non-irritant, but may cause sensitivity in some

74-MELISSA (LEMON BALM)

♦ **Attached Latin name:** *Melissa officinalis*

♦ **Applications:** allergies, insect bites, insect repellent, eczema, asthma, bronchitis, chronic coughs, colic, indigestion, nausea, menstrual problems, anxiety, depression, hypertension, insomnia, migraine, nervous tension, shock, and vertigo

◆ **Attributes:** antidepressant, antihistaminic, antispasmodic, bactericidal, carminative, cordial, diaphoretic, emmenagogue, febrifuge, hypertensive, insect repellent, nervine, sedative, stomachic, sudorific, tonic, uterine, and vermifuge

◆ **Aroma:** light, fresh, and lemony

◆ **Ably blends with:** lavender, geranium, floral, and citrus oils

◆ **Abundant areas:** native to the Mediterranean, now common throughout Europe, Middle Asia, North America, North Africa, Siberia, cultivated in France, Spain, Germany, and Russia

◆ **Acquisition:** steam distillation of leaves and flowering tops

◆ **Areas of safety:** non-toxic, but may cause sensitivity and dermal irritation | use in low dilutions only

75-MIMOSA

◆ **Attached Latin name:** *Mimosa pudica*

◆ **Applications:** oily, sensitive, general skin care, anxiety, nervous tension, over-sensitivity, and stress

◆ **Attributes:** antiseptic and astringent

♦ **Aroma:** concrete—sweet, woody, and deep floral | absolute—slightly green, woody, and floral

♦ **Ably blends with:** lavandin, lavender, ylang-ylang, violet, citronella, opopanax, Peru balsam, cassie, floral and spice oils

♦ **Abundant areas:** native to Australia, naturalized in North and Central Africa, produced in southern France and Italy

♦ **Acquisition:** concrete and absolute—solvent extraction of flowers and twig ends

♦ **Areas of safety:** non-toxic, non-irritant, and non-sensitivity

76-MINT (PEPPERMINT)

♦ **Attached Latin name:** *Mentha piperita*

♦ **Applications:** fainting, headache, mental fatigue, migraine, nervous stress, vertigo, acne, dermatitis, ringworm, scabies, toothache, colds, flu, fevers, neuralgia, muscular paint, palpitations, asthma, bronchitis, halitosis, sinusitis, spasmodic cough, colic, cramp, dyspepsia, flatulence, and nausea

♦ **Attributes:** analgesic, anti-inflammatory, antimicrobial, antiphlogistic, antipruritic, antiseptic, antispasmodic, antiviral, astringent, carminative, cephalic, cholagogue, cordial, emmenagogue, expectorant, febrifuge, hepatic, nervine, stomachic, sudorific, vasoconstrictor, and vermifuge

♦ **Aroma:** highly penetrating, grassy, minty, and camphoraceous

♦ **Ably blends with:** benzoin, rosemary, lavender, marjoram, lemon, eucalyptus, and other mints

♦ **Abundant areas:** originally, a cultivated hybrid propagated in England, naturalized throughout Europe and America, and cultivated worldwide

♦ **Acquisition:** steam distillation of the flowering herb

♦ **Areas of safety:** non-toxic, non-irritant, and non-sensitivity

77-Mint (Spearmint)

♦ **Attached Latin name:** *Mentha spicata*

♦ **Applications:** the properties resemble peppermint, but in a much more powerful way and more suited to treating children with cases of fatigue, headache, migraine, nervous strain, neurasthenia, stress, acne, dermatitis, congested skin, catarrhal conditions, sinusitis, colic, dyspepsia, flatulence, hepatobiliary disorders, nausea, vomiting, colds, fevers, and flu

♦ **Attributes:** local anesthetic, antiseptic, antispasmodic, astringent, carminative, cephalic, cholagogue, decongestant, digestive, diuretic, expectorant, febrifuge, hepatic, nervine, stimulant, stomachic, and tonic

♦ **Aroma:** warm, spicy, herbaceous, and minty

♦ **Ably blends with:** lavender, lavandin, jasmine, eucalyptus, basil, rosemary, and peppermint

♦ **Abundant areas:** native to the Mediterranean region, now common throughout Europe, Western Asia, and the Middle East

♦ **Acquisition:** steam distillation of the flowering tops

♦ **Areas of safety:** non-toxic, non-irritant, and non-sensitivity

78-MYRRH

♦ **Attached Latin name:** *Commiphora myrrha*

♦ **Applications:** athlete's foot, chapped/cracked skin, eczema, mature complexions, ringworm, wounds, wrinkles, colds, arthritis, amenorrhea, leucorrhoea, itches, thrush, asthma, bronchitis, catarrh, coughs, gum infections, gingivitis, mouth ulcers, sore throat, voice loss, diarrhea, dyspepsia, flatulence, hemorrhoids, and loss of appetite

● **Attributes:** anti-catarrhal, anti-inflammatory, antimicrobial, antiphlogistic, antiseptic, astringent, balsamic, carminative, cicatrizant, emmenagogue, expectorant, fungicidal, revitalizing, sedative, stimulant, stomachic, tonic, uterine, and vulnerary

● **Aroma:** resin—warm, rich, spicy, and balsamic | oil—warm, sweet, balsamic, slightly spicy, and medicinal

● **Ably blends with:** frankincense, sandalwood, benzoin, oakmoss, opopanax, cypress, juniper, mandarin, geranium, patchouli, mints, lavender, pine, and spice oils

● **Abundant areas:** native to North East Africa and Southwest Asia, especially in the Red Sea region

● **Acquisition:** resin absolute—solvent extraction of the crude myrrh | oil—a steam distillation of the crude myrrh

● **Areas of safety:** non-irritant and non-sensitivity, but possibly toxic in high concentrations | do not use during pregnancy

79-NARCISSUS

- **Attached Latin name:** *Narcissus poeticus*
- **Applications:** perfume
- **Attributes:** antispasmodic, aphrodisiac, emetic, narcotic, and sedative
- **Aroma:** sweet, green, and herbaceous, with a heavy floral undertone
- **Ably blends with:** clove bud, jasmine, neroli, ylang-ylang, rose, mimosa, sandalwood, Oriental and floral fragrances
- **Abundant areas:** native to the Middle East and the Eastern Mediterranean region, naturalized in Southern France, cultivated extensively for its flowers | only Holland and the Grasse region of France produce the concrete and absolute
- **Acquisition:** concrete and absolute—solvent extraction of the flowers
- **Areas of safety:** all members of this family, especially the bulbs, have a profound effect on the nervous system and can cause paralysis, and even death

80-NEROLI (BITTER ORANGE BLOSSOM)

- **Attached Latin name:** *Citrus aurantium*

♦ **Applications:** scars, stretch marks, thread veins, mature and sensitive skin, tones complexion, wrinkles, anxiety, depression, nervous tension, PMT, shock, stress-related conditions, palpitations, poor circulation, diarrhea, colic, flatulence, spasm, and nervous dyspepsia

♦ **Attributes:** antidepressant, antiseptic, antispasmodic, aphrodisiac, bactericidal, carminative, cicatrizant, cordial, deodorant, digestive, fungicidal, mild hypnotic, nervous stimulant, cardiac, and circulatory tonic

♦ **Aroma:** absolute—fresh, delicate, yet, rich, warm, sweet, and floral | oil—light sweet floral, and turpentine-like top note

♦ **Ably blends with:** absolute—jasmine, benzoin, myrrh and all citrus oils | oil—chamomile, coriander, geranium benzoin, clary sage, jasmine, lavender, opopanax, roses, ylang-ylang, lemon, and other citrus oils

♦ **Abundant areas:** native to the Far East, but well adapted to the Mediterranean climate

♦ **Acquisition:** concrete and absolute—solvent extraction of freshly picked flowers | oil—a steam distillation of freshly picked flowers

⁕ **Areas of safety:** non-toxic, non-irritant, non-sensitivity, and non-phototoxic

81-Niaouli

⁕ **Attached Latin name:** *Melaleuca quinquenervia*

⁕ **Applications:** acne, boils, burns, cuts, insect bites, oily skin, spots, ulcers, wounds, colds, fever, flu, muscular aches/pains, poor circulation, rheumatism, asthma, bronchitis, catarrhal conditions, coughs, sinusitis, sore throat, whooping cough, cystitis, and urinary infection

⁕ **Attributes:** analgesic, antihelmintic, anti-catarrhal, anti-rheumatic, antiseptic, antispasmodic, bactericidal, balsamic, cicatrizant, diaphoretic, expectorant, regulator, stimulant, and vermifuge

⁕ **Aroma:** sweet, fresh, and camphoraceous

⁕ **Ably blends with:** no data available

⁕ **Abundant areas:** native to Australia, New Caledonia, and the French Pacific Islands

⁕ **Acquisition:** steam distillation of leaves and young twigs

⁕ **Areas of safety:** non-toxic, non-irritant, and non-sensitivity

82-NUTMEG

- **Attached Latin name:** *Myristica fragrans*
- **Applications:** arthritis, gout, muscular aches/pains, poor circulation, rheumatism, flatulence, indigestion, nausea, sluggish digestion, bacterial infection, frigidity, impotence, neuralgia, and nervous fatigue
- **Attributes:** analgesic, anorexigenic, anti-emetic, anti-oxidant, anti-rheumatic, antiseptic, antispasmodic, aphrodisiac, carminative, digestive, emmenagogue, gastric secretory stimulant, larvicidal, a prostaglandin inhibitor, stimulant, and tonic
- **Aroma:** warm and spicy
- **Ably blends with:** oakmoss, lavandin, bay leaf, Peru balsam, orange, geranium, clary sage, rosemary, line, petitgrain, mandarin, coriander, and other spice oils
- **Abundant areas:** native to the Moluccas and nearby islands, cultivated in Indonesia, Sri Lanka and the West Indies, especially Granada
- **Acquisition:** steam distillation of the dried worm-eaten nutmeg seed, the dried orange-brown aril or husk (mace) | produce oleoresins in small quantities by solvent extraction from the mace

◆ **Areas of safety:** non-toxic, non-irritant, and non-sensitivity, but shows signs of toxicity in large doses | do not use during pregnancy

83-OAKMOSS

◆ **Attached Latin name:** *Evernia prunastri*
◆ **Applications:** as a fixative
◆ **Attributes:** antiseptic, demulcent, expectorant, and fixative
◆ **Aroma:** concrete and resin—heavy, rich, and tenaciously earthy | absolute—tenaciously earthy and mossy | absolute oil—dry, earthy, and bark-like
◆ **Ably blends with:** with its high fixative value, it can blend with virtually all other oils
◆ **Abundant areas:** oaks are native to Europe and North America, with its lichen collected all over Central and Southern Europe, especially France, Yugoslavia, Hungary, Greece, Morocco, and Algeria
◆ **Acquisition:** concrete and absolute—solvent extraction of the lichen | absolute oil—vacuum distillation of the concrete | resins—alcohol extraction of the raw material

♦ **Areas of safety:** extensively altered by cutting or adulteration with other lichen or synthetic perfume materials

84-OPOPANAX (HERCULES-ALL-HEAL)

♦ **Attached Latin name:** *Opopanax chironium*
♦ **Applications:** possibly similar to myrrh
♦ **Attributes:** antitoxic, antitussive, antiseptic, antispasmodic, diuretic, emmenagogue, insecticidal, nervine, rubefacient, stimulant, tonic, and vermifuge
♦ **Aroma:** liquid—sweet, balsamic, spicy, warm, and animal-like | mass—warm, powdery, sweet, balsamic, and root-like
♦ **Ably blends with:** clary sage, coriander, labdanum, bergamot, myrrh, frankincense, vetiver, sandalwood, patchouli, mimosa, fir needle, and neroli
♦ **Abundant areas:** native to East Africa and Eastern Ethiopia
♦ **Acquisition:** resin—solvent extraction of the crude oily gum resin | oil—a steam distillation of the crude oily gum resin
♦ **Areas of safety:** frequently adulterated

85-ORANGE (BITTER)

💧 **Attached Latin name:** *Citrus aurantium*

💧 **Applications:** nervous tension and stress-related conditions, obesity, palpitations, water retention, colds, flu, dull and oily complexions, mouth ulcers, constipation, dyspepsia, and spasm

💧 **Attributes:** antichlorotic, anti-inflammatory, antiseptic, astringent, bactericidal, carminative, fungicidal, mild sedative, stomachic, and tonic

💧 **Aroma:** fresh, dry, and almost floral with a rich and sweet undertone

💧 **Ably blends with:** no data available

💧 **Abundant areas:** native to the Far East, India, and China, but grows abundantly in the USA, Israel, and South America, but well adapted to the Mediterranean climate

💧 **Acquisition:** cold expression of the outer peel of the almost ripe fruit (leaves are usually for the production of petitgrain oil, and blossoms for neroli oil)

💧 **Areas of safety:** non-toxic, non-irritant, and non-sensitivity, but may be phototoxic for some

86-ORANGE (SWEET)

● **Attached Latin name:** *Citrus sinensis*
● **Applications:** nervous tension and stress-related conditions, obesity, palpitations, water retention, colds, flu, dull and oily complexions, mouth ulcers, constipation, dyspepsia, and spasms
● **Attributes:** antidepressant, anti-inflammatory, antiseptic, bactericidal, carminative, antichlorotic, digestive, fungicidal, hypotensive, nervous sedative, digestive and lymphatic stimulant, stomachic, and tonic
● **Aroma:** sweet, fresh, and fruity
● **Ably blends with:** lavender, neroli, lemon, clary sage, myrrh and spice oils such as nutmeg, cinnamon, and clove
● **Abundant areas:** native to China, cultivated in America and around the Mediterranean
● **Acquisition:** either the cold expression or steam distillation of the fresh ripe or almost ripe rinds
● **Areas of safety:** non-toxic, non-irritant, and non-sensitivity, distilled orange oil can be phototoxic

87-PALMAROSA

● **Attached Latin name:** *Cymbopogon martini*

♦ **Applications:** nervous exhaustion, stress-related conditions, acne, dermatitis, minor skin infections, scars, sores, wrinkles, all types of treatment for face, hands, feet, neck, lips, anorexia, digestive atonic, and intestinal infections

♦ **Attributes:** antiseptic, bactericidal, cicatrizant, digestive, febrifuge, hydrating, digestive and circulatory stimulant, and tonic

♦ **Aroma:** sweet, floral, rosy, and geranium-like

♦ **Ably blends with:** ylang-ylang, geranium, oakmoss, rosewood, amyris, sandalwood, guaiac wood, cedarwood, and floral oils

♦ **Abundant areas:** native to India and Pakistan, cultivated in Africa, Indonesia, Brazil, and the Comoro Islands

♦ **Acquisition:** water-steam distillation of the fresh or dried grass

♦ **Areas of safety:** non-toxic, non-irritant, and non-sensitivity

88-PARSLEY

♦ **Attached Latin name:** *Petroselinum crispum*

♦ **Applications:** amenorrhea, dysmenorrhea, labor, cystitis, urinary infection, accumulation of toxins, arthritis, broken blood vessels, cellulitis, rheumatism, sciatica, colic, flatulence, indigestion, and hemorrhoids

◆ **Attributes:** antimicrobial, anti-rheumatic, antiseptic, astringent, carminative, diuretic, depurative, emmenagogue, febrifuge, hypotensive, laxative, mild stimulant, stomachic, and uterine tonic

◆ **Aroma:** warm, woody, spicy, and herbaceous

◆ **Ably blends with:** roses, orange blossom, ylang-ylang, oakmoss, clary sage, and spice oils

◆ **Abundant areas:** native to the Mediterranean region, cultivated in California, Germany, France, Belgium Hungary, and parts of Asia

◆ **Acquisition:** steam distillation of the seed and herb

◆ **Areas of safety:** moderately toxic and irritant | used in moderation | do not use during pregnancy

89-PATCHOULI

◆ **Attached Latin name:** *Pogostemon cablin*

◆ **Applications:** acne, athlete's foot, cracked and chapped skin, dandruff, dermatitis, eczema, fungal infections, hair care, impetigo, insect repellent, sores, oily hair/skin, open pores, wounds, wrinkles, frigidity, nervous exhaustion, and stress-related complains

♦ **Attributes:** antidepressant, anti-inflammatory, anti-emetic, antimicrobial, antiphlogistic, antiseptic, antitoxic, antiviral, aphrodisiac, astringent, bactericidal, carminative, cicatrizant, deodorant, digestive, diuretic, febrifuge, fungicidal, nervine, prophylactic, nervous stimulant, stomachic, and tonic

♦ **Aroma:** sweet, rich, herbaceous, and earthy

♦ **Ably blends with:** clary sage, myrrh, cassia, bergamot, neroli, roses, lavender, clove, geranium, oakmoss, opopanax, cedarwood, sandalwood, vetiver, and labdanum

♦ **Abundant areas:** native to tropical Asia, Indonesia, and the Philippines, cultivated for its oil in India, China, Malaysia, and South America

♦ **Acquisition:** steam distillation of the dried leaves

♦ **Areas of safety:** non-toxic, non-irritant, and non-sensitivity

90-Pepper (Black)

♦ **Attached Latin name:** *Piper nigrum*

♦ **Applications:** chilblains, anemia, arthritis, muscular aches and pains, neuralgia, poor circulation, poor muscle tone, rheumatic pain, sprains, stiffness, catarrh, chills, colic, constipation, diarrhea, flatulence, heartburn, loss of appetite, nausea, colds, flu, infections, and viruses

💧 **Attributes:** analgesic, antimicrobial, antiseptic, antispasmodic, antitoxic, aperitif, aphrodisiac, bactericidal, carminative, diaphoretic, digestive, diuretic, febrifuge, laxative, rubefacient, nervous, circulatory and digestive stimulant, stomachic, and tonic

💧 **Aroma:** fresh, dry, woody, warm, and spicy

💧 **Ably blends with:** frankincense, sandalwood, lavender, rosemary, marjoram, spices, and florals oils

💧 **Abundant areas:** native to Southwest India, cultivated extensively in tropical countries

💧 **Acquisition:** oleoresin—solvent extraction, mainly for use as flavoring | oil—a steam distillation of the dried and crushed black peppercorns

💧 **Areas of safety:** non-toxic and non-sensitivity, but may be an irritant in high concentrations | use in moderation

91-PETITGRAIN

💧 **Attached Latin name:** *Citrus aurantium ssp. amara*

♦ **Applications:** convalescence, insomnia, nervous exhaustion, stress-related conditions, acne, excessive perspiration, greasy skin and hair, toning, dyspepsia, and flatulence

♦ **Attributes:** antiseptic, antispasmodic, deodorant, digestive, nervine, digestive and nervous stimulant, stomachic, and tonic

♦ **Aroma:** fresh, floral, and citrus with a woody and herbaceous undertone

♦ **Ably blends with:** rosemary, lavender, geranium, bergamot, bitter orange, orange blossom, labdanum, oakmoss, clary sage, jasmine, benzoin, palmarosa, clove, and balsams

♦ **Abundant areas:** native to Southern China and Northeast India

♦ **Acquisition:** steam distillation of the leaves and twigs

♦ **Areas of safety:** non-toxic, non-irritant, non-sensitivity, and non-phototoxic

92-PINE (SCOTCH PINE)

♦ **Attached Latin name:** *Pinus sylvestris*

♦ **Applications:** arthritis, gout, muscular aches and pains, poor circulation, rheumatism, cystitis, urinary infection, fatigue, nervous exhaustion and stress-related conditions, neuralgia, colds, flu, cuts, lice, excessive perspiration, scabies, sores, asthma, and bronchitis

♦ **Attributes:** antimicrobial, anti-neuralgic, anti-rheumatic, antiscorbutic, pulmonary, urinary and hepatic antiseptic, antiviral, bactericidal, balsamic, cholagogue, deodorant, diuretic, expectorant, hypertensive, insecticidal, restorative, rubefacient, adrenal cortex, circulatory, nervous stimulant, and vermifuge

♦ **Aroma:** strong, dry, balsamic, and turpentine-like

♦ **Ably blends with:** cedarwood, rosemary, sage, lavender, juniper, lemon, niaouli, eucalyptus, and marjoram

♦ **Abundant areas:** native to Eurasia, cultivated in the Eastern USA, Europe, Russia, the Baltic States, and Scandinavia

♦ **Acquisition:** dry distillation of the needles | steam distillation of the oleoresin produces gum turpentine

♦ **Areas of safety:** non-toxic and non-irritant, but may cause sensitivity | avoid in allergic skin conditions

93-ROSE (CABBAGE)

♦ **Attached Latin name:** *Rosa centifolia*

♦ **Applications:** broken capillaries, conjunctivitis, dry skin, eczema, herpes, mature and sensitive complexions, wrinkles, palpitations, poor circulation, asthma, coughs, hay fever, cholecystitis, liver congestions, nausea, irregular menstruation, leucorrhoea, menorrhagia, uterine, disorders, depression, impotence, insomnia, frigidity, headache, nervous tension, and stress-related disorders

♦ **Attributes:** antichlorotic, antidepressant, antiphlogistic, antiseptic, antispasmodic, anti-tubercular agent, antiviral, aphrodisiac, astringent, bactericidal, cicatrizant, depurative, emmenagogue, hemostatic, hepatic, laxative, appetite regulator, nervous sedative, stomachic, and tonic

♦ **Aroma:** oil—deep, sweet, rosy and floral absolute—deep, rich, sweet, rosy, spicy, and honey-like

♦ **Ably blends with:** jasmine, cassie, mimosa, orange blossom, geranium bergamot, lavender, clary sage, sandalwood, guaiac wood, patchouli, benzoin, chamomile, Peru balsam, clove, and Palmarosa

♦ **Abundant areas:** native to Persia, cultivated in Morocco, Tunisia, Italy, France, Yugoslavia, and China

◆ **Acquisition:** concrete and absolute—solvent extraction of the fresh petals | oil—steam-water distillation of the fresh petals

◆ **Areas of safety:** non-toxic, non-irritant, and non-sensitivity

94-ROSE (DAMASK)

◆ **Attached Latin name:** *Rosa damascena*

◆ **Applications:** broken capillaries, conjunctivitis, dry skin, eczema, herpes, mature and sensitive complexions, wrinkles, palpitations, poor circulation, asthma, coughs, hay fever, cholecystitis, liver congestions, nausea, irregular menstruation, leucorrhoea, menorrhagia, uterine, disorders, depression, impotence, insomnia, frigidity, headache, nervous tension, and stress-related disorders

◆ **Attributes:** antidepressant, antiphlogistic, antiseptic, antispasmodic, anti-tubercular agent, antiviral, aphrodisiac, astringent, bactericidal, antichlorotic, cicatrizant, depurative, emmenagogue, hemostatic, hepatic, laxative, appetite regulator, nervous sedative, stomachic, and tonic

◆ **Aroma:** essential oil—deep, rich, sweet, floral, and slightly spicy| absolute—tenaciously rich, sweet, spicy, and floral

◆ **Ably blends with:** most oils, and is useful for *'rounding off'* (balancing) blends

◆ **Abundant areas:** native to the Orient, similar types grow in China, India, and Russia, cultivated in Bulgaria, Turkey, and France

◆ **Acquisition:** concrete and absolute—solvent extraction of the fresh petals | oil—water or steam distillation of the fresh petals

◆ **Areas of safety:** non-toxic, non-irritant, and non-sensitivity

95-ROSEMARY

◆ **Attached Latin name:** *Rosmarinus officinalis*

◆ **Applications:** acne, dermatitis, dandruff, eczema, greasy hair, insect repellent, promotes hair growth, regulates seborrhea, scabies, stimulates scalp, lice, varicose veins, arteriosclerosis, fluid retention, gout, muscular pain, palpitations, poor circulation, rheumatism, asthma, bronchitis, whooping cough, colitis, dyspepsia, flatulence, hypercholesterolemia, jaundice, dysmenorrhea, leucorrhoea, colds, flu, infections, debility, neuralgia, mental fatigue, nervous exhaustion, and stress-related disorders

💧 **Attributes:** analgesic, antimicrobial, anti-oxidant, anti-parasitic, anti-rheumatic, antiseptic, antispasmodic, aphrodisiac, astringent, carminative, cephalic, cytophylactic, diaphoretic, digestive, diuretic, emmenagogue, fungicidal, hepatic, hypertensive, nervine, restorative, rubefacient, circulatory/adrenal cortex, hepatobiliary stimulant, stomachic, sudorific, tonic, and vulnerary

💧 **Aroma:** strong, fresh, minty, and herbaceous with a woody and balsamic undertone

💧 **Ably blends with:** lavender, lavender, lavandin, citronella, oregano, pine, basil, peppermint, elemi, labdanum, cedarwood, petitgrain, cinnamon, and other spice oils

💧 **Abundant areas:** native to the Mediterranean region, cultivated in California, Russia, Middle East, England, France, Spain, Portugal, Yugoslavia, Morocco, and China

💧 **Acquisition:** steam distillation of the fresh flowering tops or the whole plant

💧 **Areas of safety:** non-toxic, non-irritant, and non-sensitivity | do not use if epileptic | do not use during pregnancy

96-Rosewood (Brazilian Rosewood)

● **Attached Latin name:** *Dalbergia nigra*

● **Applications:** acne, dermatitis, scars, wounds, wrinkles, and general skin care, colds, coughs, fever, infections, stimulates the immune system, frigidity, headaches nausea, nervous tension, and stress-related conditions

● **Attributes:** mild analgesic, anticonvulsant, antidepressant, antimicrobial, antiseptic, aphrodisiac, bactericidal, cellular stimulant, cephalic, deodorant, immune system stimulant, tissue regenerator, and tonic

● **Aroma:** sweet, woody, and floral with a spicy hint

● **Ably blends with:** citrus, woods, and florals, but blends well with most oils

● **Abundant areas:** native to the Amazon region, produced by Brazil and Peru

● **Acquisition:** steam distillation of the wood chippings

● **Areas of safety:** non-toxic, non-irritant, and non-sensitivity

97-SAGE (CLARY)

💧 **Attached Latin name:** *Salvia sclarea*

💧 **Applications:** acne, boils, dandruff, hair loss, inflamed conditions, oily skin and hair, ophthalmic, ulcers, wrinkles, amenorrhea, labor pain, dysmenorrhea, leucorrhoea, high blood pressure, muscular aches and pains, frigidity, impotence, migraine, nervous tension, stress-related disorders, asthma, throat infections, whooping coughs, colic, cramp, dyspepsia, and flatulence

💧 **Attributes:** anticonvulsive, antidepressant, antiphlogistic, antiseptic, antispasmodic, aphrodisiac, astringent, bactericidal, carminative, cicatrizant, deodorant, digestive, emmenagogue, hypotensive, nervine, regulator, sedative, stomachic, and uterine tonic

💧 **Aroma:** sweet, nutty, and herbaceous

💧 **Ably blends with:** citrus oils, bergamot, frankincense, jasmine, labdanum, cedarwood, opopanax, pine, geranium, sandalwood, cardamom, coriander, lavender, and juniper

💧 **Abundant Areas:** native to Southern Europe, cultivated in the Mediterranean region, Russia, and the USA

⚫ **Acquisition:** steam distillation of the flowering tops and leaves

⚫ **Areas of safety:** non-toxic, non-irritant, and non-sensitivity | do not use during pregnancy | do not use while drinking alcohol as it can exaggerate the effects

98-Sage (Spanish)

⚫ **Attached Latin name:** *Salvia lavandulifolia*

⚫ **Applications:** acne, cuts, dandruff, dermatitis, eczema, excessive sweating, hair loss, gingivitis, gum infections, sores, headaches, nervous exhaustion, stress-related conditions, arthritis, debility, fluid retention, muscular aches and pains, poor circulation, rheumatism, jaundice, liver congestion, amenorrhea, dysmenorrhea, sterility, asthma, coughs, laryngitis, colds, fevers, and flu

⚫ **Attributes:** antidepressant, anti-inflammatory, antimicrobial, antiseptic, antispasmodic, astringent, carminative, deodorant, depurative, digestive, emmenagogue, expectorant, febrifuge, hypotensive, nervine, regulatory, stimulant, stomachic, and general tonic

⚫ **Aroma:** fresh, herbaceous, camphoraceous, and slightly pine-like

◆ **Ably blends with:** cedarwood, clary sage, juniper, citronella, eucalyptus, lavandin, lavender, rosemary, and pine-like oils

◆ **Abundant areas:** native to the mountainous regions in Spain, grows in Southwest France and Yugoslavia

◆ **Acquisition:** steam distillation of the leaves

◆ **Areas of safety:** non-toxic, non-irritant, and non-sensitivity | do not use during pregnancy | use in moderation

99-SANDALWOOD

◆ **Attached Latin name:** *Santalum album*

◆ **Applications:** acne, dry, cracked and chapped skin, aftershave, greasy skin, moisturizer, cystitis, depression, insomnia, nervous tensions, stress-related complains, bronchitis, catarrh, coughs, laryngitis, sore throat, diarrhea, and nausea

◆ **Attributes:** antidepressant, antiphlogistic, urinary and pulmonary antiseptic, antispasmodic, aphrodisiac, astringent, bactericidal, carminative, cicatrizant, diuretic, expectorant, fungicidal, insecticidal, sedative, and tonic

◆ **Aroma:** deep, soft, sweet, woody, and balsamic

♦ **Ably blends with:** violet, roses, tuberose, clove, black pepper, bergamot, rosewood, geranium, labdanum, oakmoss, benzoin, vetiver, patchouli, mimosa, cassie, costus, jasmine, myrrh, and lavender

♦ **Abundant areas:** native to tropical Asia, Sri Lanka, India, Malaysia, Indonesia, and Taiwan

♦ **Acquisition:** water or steam distillation of the powdered and dried roots and heartwood

♦ **Areas of safety:** non-toxic, non-irritant, and non-sensitivity

100-YLANG-YLANG (CANANGA)

♦ **Attached Latin name:** *Cananga odorata*
♦ **Applications:** insect bites, fragrance, general skin care, anxiety, depression, nervous tension, and stress-related problems
♦ **Attributes:** antiseptic, antidepressant, aphrodisiac, hypotensive, nervine, sedative, and tonic
♦ **Aroma:** tenaciously sweet, floral, and balsamic
♦ **Ably blends with:** birch tar, copaiba balsam, labdanum, neroli, oakmoss, jasmine, guaiac wood, and Oriental-type bases
♦ **Abundant areas:** native to tropical Asia, Java, Malaysia, the Philippines, and the Moluccas Islands

- **Acquisition:** water distillation of the flower petals
- **Areas of safety:** non-toxic, non-irritant, and non-sensitivity

NOTE: Among these essential oils, only ***ylang-ylang***, ***roses***, ***rosemary***, ***palmarosa***, ***orange***, ***lavender***, ***geranium***, ***frankincense***, ***neroli***, ***chamomile***, and ***bergamot*** oils are safe to use for children and babies.

You may find that some of your favorite essential oils are absent in the list. Similar to certain plants, you must avoid a few essential oils since some of their predominant compounds are highly toxic, if not unpleasant-smelling; and thus, they are not suitable for ideal aromatherapy practices.

Furthermore, many of them may cause further skin issues upon contact or may even be poisonous. For your guidance, the following is a list of essential oils you should avoid in aromatherapy:

- ***Yellow Camphor***
- ***Wormwood***
- ***Wormseed***

- ☠ Wintergreen
- ☠ Violet
- ☠ Vetiver
- ☠ Verbena
- ☠ Vanilla
- ☠ Turpentine
- ☠ Turmeric
- ☠ Thyme
- ☠ Thuja
- ☠ Tea Tree
- ☠ Tarragon
- ☠ Tansy
- ☠ Southernwood
- ☠ Savine
- ☠ Sassafras
- ☠ Rue
- ☠ Pennyroyal
- ☠ Oregano
- ☠ Mustard
- ☠ Mugwort
- ☠ Jaborandi leaf
- ☠ Horseradish
- ☠ Calamus
- ☠ Boldo leaf
- ☠ Bitter Almond

Glossary Guide

💧 **Abortifacient** – causing abortion

💧 **Amebicidal** – destructive to amebae

💧 **Analgesic** – an agent that reduces or eliminates pain

💧 **Anodyne** – capable of soothing or eliminating pain

💧 **Anorexigenic** – causing loss of appetite

💧 **Anti-catarrhal** – efficacious against catarrh—discharge of mucus associated with inflammation of mucous membranes, especially of the nose and throat

💧 **Antichlorotic** – treatment of iron-deficiency anemia

💧 **Anticonvulsive** – agent that prevents or relieves convulsions

💧 **Antihelmintic** – destructive to parasitic worms

💧 **Antihemorrhagic** – tending to stop the hemorrhage

💧 **Anti-hypocholesterolemia** – reduce the presence of abnormally small amounts of cholesterol in the circulating blood

💧 **Anti-neuralgic** – an agent that relieves burning nerve pains

💧 **Antiphlogistic** – reducing inflammation or fever

- **Anti-putrescent** – prevents decomposition or rotting from the breakdown of organic matters, usually by the bacterial action
- **Antiscorbutic** – preventing or curing scurvy
- **Antiseborrheic** – preventing or relieving excessive secretion of sebum or preventing or relieving seborrheic dermatitis
- **Antispasmodic** – preventing or relieving muscle spasms or cramps
- **Aperient** – gently stimulating evacuation of the bowels
- **Bactericidal** – destructive to bacteria
- **Balsamic** – relating to fragrant balsams
- **Carminative** – relieving flatulence
- **Cephalic** – pertaining to the head, or to the head end of the body
- **Cholagogue** – an agent that stimulates gallbladder contraction to promote bile flow
- **Cicatrizant** – healing or healed by the formation of scar tissue
- **Cytophylactic** – increase in cellular activity
- **Demulcent** – soothing or relieving irritation
- **Depurative** – purgative or capable of purifying
- **Diaphoretic** – an agent that promotes sweating; also called **sudorific**

◆ **Diuretic** – an agent that promotes the increase of urine extraction

◆ **Emmenagogue** – an agent that hastens or induces menstrual flow

◆ **Expectorant** – an agent that promotes the ejection of mucus or bronchial excretions from the respiratory tract by decreasing its viscosity

◆ **Febrifuge** – an agent that reduces fever; also called **antipyretic**

◆ **Galactagogic** – inducing lactation; also, lactogenic

◆ **Heartwood** – the central mass of wood in trees in which there are no living cells

◆ **Hemostatic** – acting to arrest bleeding or hemorrhage

◆ **Hepatic** – relating to the liver and its functions

◆ **Hepatobiliary** – pertaining to or emanating from the liver, bile ducts, and gallbladder

◆ **Hypoglycemic** – an agent that lowers blood glucose levels

◆ **Hypotensive** – characterized by or causing diminished tension or pressure

◆ **Larvicidal** – destructive to the larvae of insects

- **Leukocytosis** – actual increase in the total number of leukocytes in the blood, as distinguished from a relative increase (e.g., in dehydration)
- **Lipolytic** – hydrolyzing of fats and result in the production of carboxylic acids and glycerol
- **Mucolytic** – the process of breaking down mucus
- **Nervine** – a medical preparation that reduces anxiety and tension, and stimulates or strengthen the neural function
- **Ophthalmic** – pertaining to the eye
- **Parturient** – relating to or in the process of childbirth
- **Prophylactic** – an agent that acts to prevent a disease
- **Prostaglandin** – potent hormone-like compounds composed of essential fatty acids that stimulate the muscles of the uterus and affect the blood vessels; used to induce abortion or birth
- **Rubefacient** – causing redness of the skin
- **Sialagogue** – an agent that stimulates the flow of saliva
- **Soporific** – causing or producing deep sleep
- **Spasmolytic** – an agent that relieves smooth muscle spasms

◆ **Stomachic** – an agent that stimulates gastric activity

◆ **Styptic** – an agent that arrest hemorrhage with an astringent quality

◆ **Sudorific** – an agent that promotes sweating

◆ **Tonic** – invigorating; increasing physical or mental tone or strength

◆ **Vasoconstrictive** – causing the narrowing of the blood vessels

◆ **Vasodilatory** – relating to the dilation of blood vessels

◆ **Vermifuge** – destructive to parasitic worms; also called **antihelmintic**

◆ **Vulnerary** – an agent that promotes the healing of wounds

BOOK-II
Recommended Remedy Recipes

Chapter 4 - Attars for Ailments

With a potpourri of numerous ailments for which essential oils can complementarily serve a powerful natural healing process, here is a quick summary guide for facilitating your preferred picks and the recommended aromatherapy oils to use for dealing with and healing the most common ailments:

♦ **Acne** – Citruses, Mints, Niaouli, Sages, Bergamot, Camphor, Cedarwood, German Chamomile, Linaloe, Geranium, Lavender, Lemongrass, Patchouli, Rosewood, Rosemary, Sandalwood, Palmarosa

♦ **Addiction (Smoking)** – Black Pepper, Bergamot, Grapefruit

♦ **Allergy** – Roman Chamomile, Lavender, Lemon, Eucalyptus, Helichrysum, Peppermint, Sandalwood, Frankincense

♦ **Appetite Stimulation** – Aniseed, Garlic, Ginger, Orange

- **Arthritis** – Benzoin, Fennel, Juniper, Lemon, Marjoram, Chamomile, Lavender, Lovage, Rosemary
- **Asthma** – Bergamot, Cedarwood, Chamomile, Cypress, Hyssop
- **Bad Breath | Halitosis** – Myrrh, Peppermint
- **Bleeding** - Clary Sage, Cistus, Lemon, Helichrysum
- **Blisters** – Lavender
- **Bruises** – Chamomile, Lavender, Helichrysum, Cypress, Lemongrass, Geranium
- **Bronchitis** – Eucalyptus, Fennel, Hyssop Pine, Myrrh, Sandalwood
- **Burns** – Lavender, Sage, Pine, Juniper, Eucalyptus, Chamomile
- **Cellulite** – Grapefruit, Lemon, Lime, Mandarin, Fennel, Juniper, Rosemary, White Birch
- **Catarrh** – Eucalyptus, Pine, Myrrh, Sandalwood, Fennel
- **Chills** – Benzoin, Frankincense, Myrrh
- **Colds** – Eucalyptus, Lemon, Pine, Cajeput, Hyssop, Clary Sage
- **Colic** – Bergamot, Cedarwood, Chamomile, Cypress, Hyssop, Cajeput
- **Coughs** – Eucalyptus, Pine, Myrrh, Sandalwood, Fennel

♦ **Cystitis** – Bergamot, Chamomile, Sandalwood

♦ **Dandruff** – Cajeput, Cedarwood, Eucalyptus, Lavender, Patchouli, Rosemary, Clary Sage

♦ **Diarrhea** – Peppermint

♦ **Deodorant** – Bergamot, Cypress, Lemongrass, Juniper, Lavender, Sage

♦ **Depression** – Lemon, Lavender, Neroli, Tangerine

♦ **Eczema** – Geranium, Chamomile, Lavender, Bergamot, Juniper

♦ **Feet (Aching & Tired)** – Lavender, Marjoram, Peppermint

♦ **Feet (Sweaty)** – Bergamot, Clary Sage, Cypress, Lemongrass, Juniper, Lavender, Sage

♦ **Fever** – Angelica, Basil, Eucalyptus, Lemon, Peppermint, Sage, Lemongrass

♦ **Flatulence** – Angelica, Basil, Chamomile, Fennel, Peppermint, Anise

♦ **Fleas (Pets)** – Cedarwood, Lavender

♦ **Flu** – Eucalyptus, Lemon, Pine, Cajeput, Hyssop, Sage

♦ **Frigidity | Impotence** – Cedarwood, Clary Sage, Jasmine, Neroli, Patchouli, Rose, Sandalwood, Ylang-Ylang, Basil, Cinnamon, Clove, Geranium

◆ **Hair (Damaged)** – Cedarwood, Juniper, Rosemary

◆ **Gingivitis** – Eucalyptus, Lemon, Pine, Cajeput, Hyssop, Sage

◆ **Gout** – Fennel, Juniper, Lemon, Lovage

◆ **Hangover** – Fennel, Juniper

◆ **Headaches | Migraine** – Lavender, Marjoram, Peppermint

◆ **Head (Lice)** – Lavender

◆ **Hepatic Intoxication | Liver Issues** – Carrot, Black Pepper, Celery

◆ **Hypertension (High Blood Pressure)** – Lavender, Marjoram, Ylang-Ylang, Clary Sage, Jasmine, Melissa, Rose

◆ **Hypotension (Low Blood Pressure & Poor Circulation)** – Eucalyptus, Peppermint, Rosemary, Sage, Cinnamon, Clove, Black Pepper, Hyssop, Juniper

◆ **Indigestion** – Aniseed, Chamomile, Fennel, Peppermint, Caraway, Cinnamon, Melissa

◆ **Insect Bites | Stings** – Eucalyptus, Lavender, Clove, Lemon, Sage

◆ **Insect Repellents** – Cedarwood, Geranium, Citronella, Jasmine, Lavender, Lemon, Patchouli, Rosemary, Camphor, Clove, Garlic, Eucalyptus

- **Inflammatory Diseases Symptoms** – Eucalyptus, Frankincense, Lavender, Geranium, Ginger, Basil
- **Insomnia** – Bergamot, Chamomile, Lavender, Rose, Sandalwood, Sweet Marjoram, Hops, Melissa, Juniper
- **Itches** – Rose, Bergamot, Myrrh, Patchouli, Frankincense, Peppermint, Helichrysum, Eucalyptus, Chamomile
- **Jetlag** – Peppermint
- **Menstruation-Cramps (Dysmenorrhea)** – Clary Sage, Chamomile, Jasmine, Lavender, Sweet Marjoram, Cypress, Geranium
- **Menstruation-Excessive Flow (Menorrhagia)** – Clary Sage, Frankincense, Jasmine, Rose, Melissa, Myrrh
- **Menstruation-Lack of Periods (Amenorrhea)** – Chamomile, Fennel, Hyssop, Juniper, Peppermint, Sweet Marjoram
- **Menstruation (PMT)** – Clary Sage, Frankincense, Jasmine, Rose, Melissa, Myrrh
- **Motion Sickness** – Bergamot, Black Pepper, Cardamom, Coriander, Dill, Fennel, Frankincense, German Chamomile

- **Muscle Stiffness** – Black Pepper, Juniper, Rosemary, Camphor, Sweet Marjoram
- **Nausea** – Basil, Chamomile, Fennel, Peppermint, Ginger, Lemon, Cardamom
- **Nervous Conditions | Tension** – Chamomile, Clary Sage, Juniper, Lavender, Rosemary, Ylang-Ylang, Basil, Bergamot, Marjoram, Neroli, Sandalwood
- **Obesity** – Grapefruit, Lemon, Lime, Mandarin, Fennel, White Birch
- **Pains | Aches** – Peppermint, Lavender, Clary Sage, Eucalyptus, Rosemary, Juniper
- **Rheumatism** – Black Pepper, Juniper, Rosemary, Camphor, Eucalyptus, Sweet Marjoram
- **Scar Tissues** – Chamomile, Geranium, Lavender, Rose, Frankincense, Neroli
- **Sinusitis** – Eucalyptus, Pine, Myrrh, Sandalwood, Basil, Fennel, Peppermint
- **Skin (Dermatitis)** – Benzoin, Geranium, Juniper, Lavender
- **Skin (Dry)** –Geranium, Sandalwood
- **Skin (Oily)** – Grapefruit, Lemon, Lime
- **Skin (Sweaty)** – Clary Sage, Cypress, Eucalyptus, Lemon, Lavender
- **Sore-Throat** –Eucalyptus, Lemon, Pine, Cajeput, Hyssop, Sage

- **Spots (Aging Signs & Wrinkles)** – Lavender, Geranium, Eucalyptus, Lemon, Clary Sage, Roman Chamomile, Frankincense, Myrrh, Helichrysum, Rosemary
- **Sprain |Twists** – Chamomile (German or Moroccan), Cypress, Eucalyptus, Geranium, Lavender, Sweet Marjoram, Pine, Rosemary
- **Stress** – Geranium, Jasmine, Lavender, Marjoram, Ylang-Ylang, Pine, Rose
- **Stretch Marks** – Chamomile, Geranium, Lavender, Rose, Frankincense, Lemongrass, Neroli
- **Sun Burn (Mild)** – Chamomile, Lavender
- **Swellings | Sores** – Lemongrass, Arnica, Cypress, Lemon
- **Tantrums** – Chamomile, Lavender
- **Travel Sickness** – Ginger
- **Varicose Veins** – Cypress, Lemon
- **Water Retention** – Grapefruit, Lemon, Lime, Mandarin, Fennel, White Birch
- **Weakness | Fatigue | Lethargy (Lack of Mental or Physical Strength)** – Basil, Rosemary, Peppermint, Lemon
- **Weight Issues-Excessive** – Grapefruit, Cinnamon, Ginger, Lemon, Bergamot, Peppermint, Fennel

◆ **Wounds | Abrasions | Cuts | Scrapes | Slits** – Lavender, Rosemary, Myrrh, Helichrysum, Geranium

Advised Applications

The summary guideline of recommended aromatherapy oils for dealing with and treating an ailment comes along their advisable applications. Generally, you will only have a choice of the following:

◆ **Diffusing them into the atmosphere**—follow the recommended oil drop capacities of your aromatherapy lamp or diffuser

◆ **Combining them in skin care, bath, and spa items**—creams, balms, ointments, lotions, liniments, soaps, and shampoos, etc. to enhance these products

◆ **Applying them topically to the skin**—only when diluted with water, base oil, or carrier with a recommended blend of 2-drops of an essential oil to 1-tsp of carrier oil (for further measurement conversions: 1-tsp=100 drops; 2-tsp=1-tbsp=0.5 fl. oz.)

⚫ **Spraying them into the atmosphere**—either in diluted form or using their hydrosol version

⚫ **Inhaling them directly**—from a piece of the oil-soaked cotton ball or oil-dropped tissue paper, or straight from the container

⚫ **Placing them in a nasal inhaler**—with an advisable number of drops not to exceed 15-drops

⚫ **Absorbing them into a cloth for either a hot or a cold compress**—by adding 5-drops of an essential oil to 1-cup of cold/warm water

Chapter 5 - Wellness & Welfare

Anxiety Alleviation & Nixing Nervousness

Several aromatherapy oils serve satisfactorily to relieve feelings of anxieties. Among them are lavender, jasmine, basil, bergamot, chamomile, rose, ylang-ylang, frankincense, clary sage, patchouli, geranium, marjoram, and fennel. You only have to inhale any of your preferred oils directly, or add them in a diffuser or diluted solution of a warm bath.

Although many studies show that aromatherapy could help to relieve anxiety, there is still no substitute for seeing your physician. An aromatherapy session or two might be necessary if you become anxious about meeting schedules or have a stressful day at work.

Creativity & Concentration

♦ **<u>Focus Facilitator:</u>** Use this massage blend to facilitate creative work and enhance concentration. Mix 3-drops each of clary sage and bergamot oils with 1-tbsp grapeseed oil (or any carrier oil you choose). Place 1 or

2 drops of the blend on your fingertips and gently massage your temples. Close your eyes; take a deep breath as the warm and sweet fragrance of the blend settles in to refocus and relax you.

Stress Supervision

Stress results from many issues of daily living. The following are natural recipes to help you deal with stress and prevent a regular stress from intensifying into a more debilitating chronic stress condition:

♦ **<u>Insomnia-Influenced Stress Solver:</u>** Blend 7-drops of clary sage, 4-drops of lemon, and 6-drops of lavender oil to 1-fl. oz. (30ml) almond oil. Rub a few drops of the blend between your palms and deeply inhale the aroma. Subsequently, massage your temples and nape with the blend. Visualize tranquil and relaxing scenes and feel the tension liberate from your system.

♦ **<u>Emotionally Experienced Stress Solver:</u>** For all types of emotional stress, resolve them by blending 3-drops of chamomile to 4-drops of lavender oils. Pour the blend into your bath water and soak in the tub or simply inhale the blend.

♦ **Mentally Maladjusted Stress Solver:** Mix 2-drops of peppermint with 4-drops of lavender oil and add the blend in your bath or use it in a diffuser.

Fighting Fatigue & Leaving Lethargy

♦ **Massage Mix for Enduring Energy:** A highly uplifting blend, this is great for combating lethargy or needing a pick-me-up to maintain focus and clarity. Mix 20-drops each of peppermint and spearmint, 35-drops of lavender, and 25-drops of lemon oils in a bottle. Shake well before using.

To apply, add 3 drops of the blend to 1-oz. sweet almond oil (or your preferred carrier oil). Place a few drops to your fingertips and massage gently the temples during times of confusion or stress.

You may also apply the blend by directly inhaling it from the bottle. Alternatively, you can place a few drops of the blend on your room diffuser.

Mental & Mood Melioration

♦ **Mood Makeover Mist:** Create your own all-natural body mist to spritz your face (close your eyes), your feet, hands, arms, etc. to evoke the moods you desire. Mix 6 drops ylang-ylang, 5 drops rose attar and 1-drop clove bud with 1-cup of water in a mister. Essential oils float on water; hence, do not forget to shake well before each use.

♦ **Muster Mental Functions & Facility:** To enhance your mental faculties, mix 2-drops each of neroli and lavender oils with 1-drop each of sandalwood, ylang-ylang, and jasmine oils, and add the blend to your diffuser. Diffuse it during times when you usually exercise your mental functions most.

Motion Malady

♦ **Streetwalker Spritzer:** This recipe contains oils that are relaxing, refreshing, and producing a total balancing effect to diffuse stress on the road. Mix 2-drops each of clary sage, geranium, and peppermint oil with 6-drops lavender oil and 2-oz. water in a spray bottle. Shake before applying 2-3 sprays in your car's interiors.

Insomnia Issues & Slumber Stumpers

♦ **Perfumed Pillow Plugin:** As a part of your bedtime ritual, use lavender oil for its calming and relaxing properties. Make a lavender-scented pillow insert by adding 3-drops of lavender oil to a linen square or washcloth and inserting it in your pillowcase.

- **Snore-Silencing Solution:** For a relaxing slumber, the easiest way to gain the benefits of a peaceful night is by placing a few drops of any of the suggested snore-silencing aromatherapy oils—lavender, marjoram, eucalyptus, pine, and lemon—to a diffuser before bedtime and heading off to dreamland.

Menstruation & Menopausal Mitigation

Consuming healthier diets high in vegetable and fiber content but free from processed foods, sugars, and trans-fats tremendously reduce menstrual issues. Regular physical exercises can help as well. Other things, like yoga and meditation, can also manage to resolve symptoms of premenstrual syndrome (PMS).

However, applying aromatherapy with the use of aromatic oils can be more instrumental in mitigating symptoms of menstrual cramps and PMS in a natural way. Lavender, rose, ylang-ylang and chamomile are the trustworthy oils to carry out the benefits.

First, you can blend these oils in equal proportions and place a few drops in a diffuser. Incidentally, this is the most popular and easiest way to administer the oils for this intent.

Second, you can also combine 2-drops of each of the oils with 2-tbsp of either an almond or coconut base oil. You rub the blend into the area where the cramps are occurring at their worst.

Depression Deferment

💧 **Lemon Lift:** With a balanced blend of relaxing and inspiring oils, this recipe provides a gentle uplifting effect on your emotions. Mix 20-drops each of lemon and tangerine oils with 25-drops of neroli and 35-drops lavender oils and store the blend in a tightly sealed container.

To apply, place a few drops on a piece of cotton ball or on your handkerchief, and inhale the aroma deeply every time you feel depressed or need a little boost. You can also use this blend in an aromatherapy lamp or diffuser.

Physical Pains & Acute Aches

Physical pains and acute aches usually constitute three typical symptoms: the pain or ache, tensions arising from feeling the pain, and a resultant swelling of the pained area. These symptoms can occur singularly, come as a couple, or manifest as a dreadful combination of the three components.

♦ **For pain relief only:** use ginger, black pepper, and clove oils.

♦ **For tension relief only:** apply clary sage and juniper oils.

♦ **For swelling relief only:** trust on lemongrass and arnica oils.

♦ **For tension and swelling reliefs only:** rely on cypress and sandalwood oils.

♦ **For pain and swelling reliefs only:** depend on lavender, eucalyptus, Roman and German chamomiles, and rosemary oils.

◆ **For a combo of pain, tension, and swelling reliefs**: muster the natural healing powers of peppermint, helichrysum, and marjoram oils.

You can use the oils separately or combine them to create your personalized blend for this intent. The recommended ratio for diluting the oils is 15-drops of the essential oil to 6-tsp of carrier oil, which include any of your choice of olive, coconut, or argan oils.

When applying the blend, it can be either massaged on the affected area or added to a tubful of water for a relaxing bath (10-12 drops). You can also apply it to a cold or warm compress by adding 15-drops of any specifically intended oil to a small bowl filled with warm water, then soaking a small towel in the bowl until fully wet.

Cold compresses are usually for soothing inflammation, while hot compresses are typically applied for relieving pain.

Leave the towel on the affected area for about 15 minutes. Repeat the procedure and reapply the compress, as necessary, throughout the day.

♦ **Aromatherapy Analgesic Basic Balm:** Blend 2-drops each of lemongrass, peppermint, and frankincense oils to 1-tbsp carrier oil of choice. Rub the blend onto pain-affected areas of your body.

Libido Lift

Stress can sometimes kill libido. However, there are also times that frigidity, or the lack of warmth, can ruin romantic desires and moments of intimacy with your partner. Have a boost of your romanticism with the magic works of the following aromatherapy aphrodisiac blends:

♦ **Aphrodisiac Attars for Sensual Settings:** Blend 6-drops of sandalwood, 4-drops of ylang-ylang, 3-drops of geranium, and 2-drops of neroli oils in a 2-oz. spray bottle, and fill it up with distilled water. Shake well to blend fully before each use. Spritz on comforters, pillows, and in the air before bedtime to promote sensuality and intimacy.

♦ **Romantic Rub:** Whip up a romantic body massage oil for your intimate moments with your mate by adding 2-drops each of sandalwood, neroli, and cinnamon oils with 6-drops of jojoba or sweet almond oil into your favorite massage lotion. Shake well before massaging on the skin.

Sustained Stoppage to Smoking

Kicking the smoking habit in the butt could require a daily dose of a healthy eating regimen, physical exercises, hydrating the body with more fluids, and meditation. Aromatherapy is not the general solution for stopping smoking; but rather, it is a sustainable aid to complement the quitting process.

⚫ **Smoker Stuff Solution:** Combine 40-drops of black pepper, 20-drops of clary sage, 30-drops of bergamot, 30-drops of grapefruit, 10-drops of Roman chamomile, 20-drops of marjoram, and 24-drops of coriander oils in a 15-mL amber glass bottle. Mix the oils by swirling gently the bottle.

You can use this blend through either an aromatherapy inhaler, through *smelling salts*, or by simply placing drops in a diffuser. When diffusing the blend, simply follow the recommended amount of oil drops for your diffuser.

When using an inhaler, place 25 to 30-drops of the blend into a small bowl. Add enough to soak the inhaler's cotton pad in the bowl, and roll it by using a pair of tweezers, never with your fingers. Place the soaked pad into your inhaler tube. Whenever you feel the urge to smoke, inhale for up to 2 minutes, which is the estimated time to take smoking a cigarette.

For combining the blend with *smelling salts*, add 30-drops of the blend in a ⅓-oz. (10-mL) glass bottle. Fill the bottle with coarse or fine salt. Take deep inhalations with the bottle under your nose while wafting it for 2-minutes.

Child Care & Toddler Temper Tantrums Tamer

If the meltdown of your sweet child starts getting you down, tame the revved-up emotions and mind to a slowdown. You need not be a clown to alter the frown, but you can rely on aromatherapy for a calming rubdown.

♦ **Child Calming Concoction:** Blend 1-drop of lavender oil to 1-tbsp of olive oil. Gently rub the blend on your child's skin, but only after testing the blend first on the inside of the elbow to ensure the blend has no reactionary effects. It can also be helpful to diffuse undiluted lavender oil in the air.

◆ **Scare Spray:** This spray's content, which should be contained in a 3.5-oz. mister is actually a neroli hydrosol. Its light, gentle, and uplifting aroma is pleasing to most children (and even adults!). Generally regarded to be safe for children's use, it has the added benefit of enhancing a sense of calmness and relaxation.

This makes for a soft and soothing aromatic playpen, where your child can play with ease. Another purpose is to let your child use the spray as a pseudo-repellent to scary thoughts about the boogeyman, gremlins, monsters, and other creepy creatures lurking under the bed or in the dark closet.

Although this intent does not suggest the real existence of these scary critters, remember that this is all about the creativity of engaging with aromatherapy. Thus, it must be lots of fun!

Not only has this spray given your child a peaceful playing space but also, a complete control over these scary imaginations. Additionally, it may help to conquer your child's anxieties and fears during bedtime. Hence, it will certainly encourage a relaxing and undisturbed sleep.

Meditation & Mindfulness

Meditation augments reaching higher levels of consciousness. However, your inner toxicities can impede the ethereal journey and snuff out your meditative states.

When you consider having a complete emotional cleansing, try turning negative vibes into positive ones. To complement this task is to bathe your spirit with a soothing aroma.

⬥ **Blissful Blend:** Combine 8-drops of frankincense, 3-drops of bergamot, and 2-drops each of Atlas cedarwood and rose oils in a small glass container. Soak a cotton pad into the blend and place it in your nasal inhaler. Inhale with deep breaths while closing your eyes for an immediate escape, entering into a mindful and meditative state.

Chapter 6 - Aesthetic Applications

Body Bulges (Cellulite Clearing | Weight Worries)

Grapefruit, cinnamon, and ginger are the top aromatherapy essential oils that help to shed off excess body weight. Others are bergamot, fennel, sandalwood, eucalyptus, lavender, orange, jasmine, frankincense, lemon, peppermint, and rosemary.

Using these aromatics for weight loss intents will primarily overcome common issues that plague many people on their weight loss journeys such as fatigue, inflammation, digestive disorders, lack of motivation, and sugar cravings. The following are some of the specific procedures of using these oils for weight loss:

♦ **Grapefruit for Weight Loss:** There are five ways to apply grapefruit oil for losing weight. First, you can drink it as soon as you wake up in the morning and after every meal by adding 1-2 drops of therapeutic-grade grapefruit oil in a glassful of water.

Second, you can inhale the oil directly from the bottle or add a few drops to a piece of cotton ball and breathe in deeply.

Third, you can apply it topically by rubbing the oil on your wrists, temples, chest, and just below your nose.

Fourth, you can place a few drops of grapefruit oil to your diffuser, especially during a craving attack or restraining late night snacking.

Lastly, you can reduce cellulite by blending 15-drops of the oil with ½-cup coconut oil. Rub and massage the blend onto areas of your skin that require firming or where the cellulite is.

♦ **Cinnamon for Weight Loss:** With a safe classification from the U.S. FDA, you can drink 100% pure cinnamon oil daily. Add 1-2 drops of therapeutic-grade cinnamon oil into a teacup with warm water and sweeten the brew with raw honey.

You can also inhale the oil directly from its bottle before every meal to reduce your craving and prevent overeating. Alternatively, you can apply it topically by combining 1-2 drops of the oil with base oil and rub the blend on your chest and wrists.

Finally, you can place a few drops of cinnamon oil to your diffuser. Its aroma not only makes your house smell great and boosts your mood but also, helps to rein in those late-night snack attacks.

♦ **<u>Ginger for Weight Loss:</u>** The FDA also classifies ginger oil as safe for internal use, but it is prudent to use the therapeutic-grade kind.

You can drink ginger oil by adding 1-2 drops of it into a glassful of warm water. For a balanced taste, add a squeeze of fresh lemon juice and raw honey.

You can also inhale the spicy aroma of the oil straight from the bottle. Its effects not only provide you with a good pick-me-up mood but also, reduce your cravings and appetite.

Facial Fixes (Acne | Age Spots | Chapped Lips | Wrinkles)

Advisable aromatherapy oils for facial care are frankincense, rosemary, lavender, clary sage, sandalwood, neroli, chamomile, juniper, cypress, lemongrass, basil, geranium, ylang-ylang, and lemon.

For your base oils, they can be a choice of the following: olive, grape seed, coconut, almond, or avocado oil.

⬥ **Acne Astringent Application:** To kill pore-blocking and acne-causing bacteria, apply 2-drops of clary sage oil diluted in 1-tsp of fractionated coconut or jojoba oil with a clean cotton ball to the area of concern.

⬥ **Age Spots & Anti-Aging Serum:** Mix 20-drops each of rose and carrot seed oils with 1-cup apricot kernel oil in an amber bottle. Massage a small amount of the blend over the face and neck and other concerned areas.

⬥ **Lip Balm for Dry, Chapped & Bleeding Lips:** Combine 4-drops of lavender oil with 2-tsp coconut oil into a lip balm container. Dab this creamy lip balm onto the lips whenever they feel uncomfortable. Symptoms will disappear within 3 days of using the balm consistently.

⬥ **Worriless Wrinkle Wax:** To tone the skin, promote new skin cell growths, and reduce wrinkle-producing skin oxidation, follow a rule of thumb for preparing a remedial solution:

⬥ **For normal skin:** Dilute 15-drops of aromatherapy essential oil per ounce of base oil

⬥ **For sensitive skin:** Dilute 6-drops of aromatherapy essential oil per ounce of base oil.

Hair Hygiene (Brittleness | Dandruff | Oiliness)

Lavender oil supports hair health when used regularly on the scalp. Rosemary oil is reliable to treat dry and brittle hair. Patchouli oil is helpful for treating a scaly and itchy scalp due to dandruff. Cedarwood combats oily hair and scalp. Use these hair essential oils with their following blends:

● **Scalp Massage Blend:** Warm ½-cup of olive oil and blend into 10-drops of lavender oil. Apply the blend to your hair by gently massaging your scalp to provide strong hair follicles and growths. Wrap a warm cloth or towel around your head. Sit back and relax for 15-20 minutes. Follow by applying your natural shampoo and conditioner.

● **Dry & Brittle Hair Conditioner Oil:** Mix 3-drops of rosemary with 1-tbsp jojoba oil or other carrier oils. Wet your hair with warm water and then apply conditioner. Let it sit on your hair for about 15 to 30 minutes before washing your hair as normal.

● **Dandruff Deterrent & Scaly Scalp Solution:** Blend 2-drops of patchouli, 2-drops of cedarwood, 2-drops rosemary, 2-drops of lavender oils to ½-oz. of base oil, preferably jojoba. Apply by placing 3-5 drops of the blend on the fingertips and massaging the scalp.

● **Oily Scalp:** Add 6-drops cedarwood, 6-drops rosemary, and 4-drops cypress oils to 50-mL of olive oil. Blend well and massage on the scalp. Leave the blend to soak overnight on the scalp. Shampoo thoroughly the following day.

Skin Supplements (Oiliness & Dryness)

Always check first with your dermatologist to ensure the oils you will be using are acceptable, especially if you have skin allergies or other medical conditions. Always use high quality and 100% pure essential oils.

Never use essential oils directly or *neat* onto your skin. Remember, when applying topically; always dilute the oil first with your preferred carrier oil (typically, 2-drops of oil in 1-tsp of carrier oil).

For oily skin, rosemary, cedarwood, fennel, and lemon oils are ideal choices. For dry skin, choose neroli, clary sage, patchouli, helichrysum, lavender, and sandalwood.

♦ **Oily Skin Cleanser:** Fill your soap dispenser with ¼-cup of liquid castile soap and ½-cup water. Add 7 to 10-drops of cedarwood oil and shake thoroughly to combine. You may also add 4-drops of geranium oil to give your cleanser a gorgeous fragrance.

♦ **Dry Skin Moisturizer:** Create a dilution of 4-drops of lavender oil and 4-tbsp of virgin coconut oil.

Massage your skin with the blend after a warm shower, which will open your pores. Leave the blend on your skin for at least 15 minutes.

◆ **Skin Cream:** Add 2-drops of rosemary oil to your daily skin cream for your protection against oxidative stress.

◆ **Calming Body Oil/Lotion:** Add 3-5 drops of lavender oil to 2 tbsp of carrier oil like jojoba oil or sweet almond to promote relaxation and skin health, especially during times of dry winter.

Soak, Soap & Shampoo

Sweet orange and rosemary oils are clarifying and refreshing scents ideal for liquid soaps and shampoos, and even household sprays.

◆ **Soap & Shampoo Strength**: To promote hair volume, clarify your hair, and increase the circulation in your scalp, add 1-2 drops of rosemary oil to your shampoo. You can also use lavender, basil, or cedarwood.

◆ **<u>Soothing Soak:</u>** Create a skin-soothing and emotionally uplifting citrus and herbal scented bath. Mix thoroughly 8-drops each of tangerine, lavender, and chamomile oil with 4-tbsp sea salt and 2-tbsp baking soda. Pour your desired amount to the bath water. To enhance skin nourishment, you may add 1-cup whole milk to the bath.

◆ **<u>Soap-making Solutions:</u>** Lavender, rosemary, lemon, cedarwood, patchouli, clary sage, sweet orange, bergamot, and cubeb oils are excellent aromatic supplements for soap making. Besides, each of them works well with each other when blending.

With these 10 oils, you will have a hundred possible combination blends at your disposal. Even if you just begin blending by using only a couple of oils evenly (1:1 ratio) in a blend, you will have 50 possible combinations; so, get your creative juices flowing! As starter blends, you can try out these following recipes:

For a smooth and lemony blend, combine into your soap solution 50% lemon, 30% rosemary, 15% cedarwood, and 5% cubeb oils.

For some herbal and citrus shades, blend into your soap mix 35% orange, 25% rosemary, 20% lavender, 15% peppermint, and 5% cubeb oils.

For a masculine touch, mix into your soap concoction 50% lavender, 20% clary sage, 10% orange, 10% patchouli, 5% cedarwood, and 5% cubeb oils.

Nail Nourishment

Myrrh, lavender, lemon, frankincense, and geranium are the prime essential oils for a healthy nail care regimen. Yet, these oils only complement to nourish your nails. You still need to do your share of properly caring for your nails such as the following: eating foods rich in omega-3 fatty acids, allowing your cuticles to grow by not cutting them, pampering them rather abusing them, and not going dehydrated.

⬥ **Strong & Shiny Nourished Nails Routine Rub:** Add 3-drops of geranium, 3-drops of lavender, and 2-drops of lemon oils with 4-tbsp of jojoba oil in a roll-on bottle. Blend thoroughly until incorporated. To use, rub onto your cuticles and nails daily at bedtime.

Chapter 7 - Hearth & Home

Candle Creations

Aromatherapy candles are wonderful for meditation, relaxation, and special occasions. Ensure the candle constitutes pure aromatherapy essential oils, organic soy or natural beeswax with a natural and non-lead wick.

Cleaning Concoctions

⬥ **Homemade Disinfectant:** Mix 15 to 20-drops of preferred essential oils (lavender, peppermint, and lemon) with 1-cup rubbing alcohol in a clean spray bottle by giving it a good shake. As soon as you spray, wipe down the surfaces with a clean piece of cloth and allow it to dry.

⬥ **Freshened Window Cleaner:** Mix 4-tbsp of vinegar with 12-drops lemon oil in a 32-oz. bottle. Fill it with water. Shake the bottle before spraying.

⬥ **Freshened Household Cleaner:** Add 2-drops of rosemary oil to your household cleaner for a freshened scent

♦ **<u>Wood Furniture Polisher:</u>** You only have five options on which essential oil to use for cleaning and polishing your wooden furniture: lemon, sweet orange, cedarwood, pine, and lavender oils. Mix ¼-cup of olive oil or any other carrier oil you prefer with ¼-cup white vinegar and 10-drops of any of the five suited aromatic oils. Shake well until combined thoroughly.

To use, simply spray onto a piece of microfiber cloth, and then, wipe down your wooden furniture. You need not use this polishing spray often; instead, use it once every 2 to 3 months.

Clothing Care

Eucalyptus or lemon oil is best in caring for your clothing or laundry. Lavender, orange, geranium, and mandarin are also great alternatives.

♦ **<u>Laundry & Linen:</u>** Only add 4-5 drops of your preferred clothing care oil into a wool dryer ball or a small rag and toss it in your washing machine dryer before switching it on.

● **Fabric Conditioner:** Add 4-6 drops into the washer during the wash cycle. Add the same amount with a little bit of water into the fabric softener compartment before starting a cycle.

Fragrant Fresheners

Eucalyptus or lemon oil is also ideal for freshening up your home. They can provide a refreshing, cleansing, and an invigorating fragrance.

● **House Freshener:** Select either one or use both by simply adding 4-drops to a diffuser.

TIP: For optimal effectiveness, use aromatherapy essential oils within a year after opening the bottle.

● **House Humidifier:** For keeping your humidifier smelling fresh, add 6-9 drops of peppermint oil.

● **Desk Diffusion:** As an all-natural alternative for the 'smelling salts,' this room freshener not only helps to train your focus on your house works but also, inspire you working amidst a fragrant space.

Mix 20-drops of lavender oil with ¼-cup coarse sea salt into a jar with a tight-fitting lid. Sprinkle the blend over petals of roses in a container and replace the lid. Add more oil when the scent eventually fades.

TIP: To facilitate aroma diffusion, place the opened jar near the fan port of your computer to let the fan function as a diffuser.

◆ **Carpet Cologne:** If your house has wall-to-wall carpeting, this gives you a brilliant advantage to freshen up its entire spaces. Add fragrance to your rooms by freshening up their respective carpets.

Mix 7-10 drops of lemon or eucalyptus oil (or your preferred oil) with1-cup cornstarch or baking soda in a large bowl. By using a fork, break up any clumps; stir well. Pour the mixture into a perforated can or a cheese shaker.

Sprinkle the mixture liberally over the carpet. Let it stand on the carpet for half an hour before vacuuming.

◆ **Fire Logs:** Place 1-drop of sandalwood, pine, cypress, or cedarwood oil on your fire logs about half an hour prior to burning them. Never use several perfumed logs at a time. Remember, a little goes a long way.

◆ **Stuffed Toys:** Soothe your kids while they play their stuffed toys with the calming scent of chamomile or lavender. Put a plastic bag inside a stuffed toy. Add a few drops of either oil. Seal the bag overnight.

The stuffed toy will have the dispersed scent the following day. The scent can last for up to a couple of weeks before reapplying.

Gardening Gear (Indoor | Outdoor)

◆ **Garden Insect Deterrent:** Add 10-drops each of clove, rosemary, basil, and peppermint oils in a 4-oz. spray bottle. Fill the spray bottle with water and shake well to combine fully. Spray on your garden plants to get rid of insects.

◆ **Pollinator Attractor Spray:** Add 6 to 8-drops of orange oil in a 4-oz. spray bottle and top off with water. Shake the blend before spraying it on buds and flowers to attract bees for their pollination.

⬥ **Plant Fungi Suppressant:** Mix 25-drops of clove oil with water in a 4-oz. spray bottle. Spray the blend on the soil and plants to help restrain growths of fungi.

⬥ **Fruit and Vegetable Wash:** Add in 6 to 8 drops of lemon or orange oil and ½-cup vinegar in a large bowl filled with cold water. Place your fruits and vegetables in the bowl to soak for about 8-10 minutes, and then, rinse well.

Rodent Repellent (Insect | Pest)

⬥ **Insect Repellent:** Add 2-drops of lavender or citronella oil on a piece of cloth or cotton ball and leave it on a table or night desk to rid moths and mosquitoes temporarily.

If applying topically, create a dilution of 2-drops of either oil with 1-tsp of carrier oil, and wipe the blend on your skin with a cotton ball. Do not throw the used cotton ball as you can also place it nearby.

⬥ **Pest Deterrent:** Mix 1-drop of peppermint oil with 10-parts water, together with a dash of your liquid dish detergent in a spray bottle. Spray it liberally around doorways and window frames to deter entry of mice, spiders, and other pests.

It is also easy to make your own natural insect repellent spray at home. Aside from peppermint oil, your top choices of aromatherapy essential oils for repelling insects at home are clove, rosemary, peppermint, lemongrass, lemon eucalyptus, geranium, citronella, cinnamon, and cedarwood.

Take note that the spray may only provide temporary relief from pests. They require higher concentrations and more frequent application than some commercial repellents.

However, you should also consider that water, high temperatures, sunscreens, evaporation from the wind, or sweat, can lower effectiveness. Hence, when making your preparations, ensure to consume only what you think is necessary.

Pet Preferences

Similar with humans, it is safe to use aromatherapy oils on your pets. However, there are recommended and restricted oils for pet care.

The top recommended oils are cedarwood, marjoram, myrrh, chamomile, lavender, and clary sage. On the contrary, the restricted oils are all citrus oils (especially if you are a cat lover), garlic, clove, and birch oils.

♦ **Favored Fragrances for Furry Favorites:** You need to perform a lot of testing before using an essential oil on your pets for a prolonged period. As a start, add 1 to 2-drops of any of the pet-friendly oils to a diffuser. Allow the aroma to permeate the area within 15-minute intervals.

Be sure of keeping your door open so your pets can easily leave the area if the aroma begins to bother them. Perform the test on the other recommended oils. Carefully monitor your pet's reactions for any approval or discomfort they may experience before applying the preferred pet oil on a regular basis.

Stench Suppression

Tangerine, sage, orange, mandarin, lime, lemongrass, lemon, lavender, grapefruit, and bergamot are reliable aromatherapy essential oils for reducing smoky, musty, and stale odors indoors.

⬥ **Indoor Ionizer:** Just place a few drops on any of these oils on your diffuser to serve as an ionizer cum deodorizer.

⬥ **Baking Soda-Based Deodorizer:** Alternatively, you can try mixing 2-cups of baking soda with 30-drops of lavender oil and apply by sprinkling it to where the stench occurs.

⬥ **Vinegar-Based Deodorizer:** Another similar formula is mixing 30-drops of any aromatic oils suitable for deodorizing with 2-tbsp of white distilled vinegar in a 4-oz. spray bottle. Fill the bottle with water and shake well until incorporated fully. Spray on areas where the bad odors emanate.

Towards Total Transformation Through Aromatherapy: A Conclusion

Indeed, scents are powerful! A trivial scent can instantly trigger recollections of a person, a place, or perhaps, a reverie. Aromas bear the power to evoke memories and summon emotions instantly. Fact is that they can influence directly our bodies through our brains, nervous system…and our entirety!

You may visualize aromatic essential oils as penetrating to the innermost sanctuaries of your soul to affect the mind, body, and spirit. Yet, it is much more profound to perceive these botanical oils as engaging directly with your spirit to create a soul-to-soul bond—between you and plants—a communion and a relationship that recognizes the essential oil as a sacred living being.

At first, you must have been unaware that you can love plants and their essential oils and nutrients. Now, it should be compelling to study more on the science of their components, the art of blending aromatic essential oils, and, know how to engage with and deal all about aromatherapy for life!

Nevertheless, aromatherapy is neither your panacea nor your doctor. It is an alternative medicine practice and a complementary process for natural healing. It taps the potent healing powers of aromas from essential oils extracted meticulously from plants so that you can attain a total balance of your mind, body, and spirit.

There is a wide world of benefits for you to gain from essential oils, as well as an equally diverse selection of these aromatic oils for your preference. They provide a natural supplement in a broad range of health issues without the several side effects, which many conventional medical options usually give.

Despite deficient proof and evidence from the medical field to support most of the healing abilities of essential oils, more and more people continue to use them today through aromatherapy. With that said, aromatherapy must be efficient and effective in transforming the lives of legions of people for the better.

Nonetheless, there will always be naysayers because they fail to realize their intents with aromatherapy. For instance, let us say you intended to use aromatherapy to shed off excessive weight. We all know that eating a balanced diet, exercising, and watching portion size, are all keys to losing weight.

However, there is not one dietary plan or weight loss program that is appropriate for all of us. Similarly, there has never been a fixed recipe concerning the blending of essential oils. What might truly work for you might not really work for someone else, and vice versa!

Therefore, since all of us are biochemically and uniquely exclusive, it is only fitting to keep on experimenting with a variety of essential oils. Listen to your body, hear its whispers, sensations, and murmurs. Find the personalized blends that work most efficiently and effectively for you!

Seriously, hitting your goals and satisfying your intents can be addictive, like the scents of aromatics, so never be surprised if you start enjoying it!

Everything goes as easy as counting 123 and reciting ABC when you have the proper focus, interest, and knack for learning something new! Introducing yourself to engage with aromatherapy is nothing different.

It seems tough at the start, but your strong resolve, intents, and willingness to learn will get you going until the end. Once aromatherapy becomes your new best friend, have fun blending and inhaling from here on!

You will notice improvements in your overall health and well-being. Fact is that you will feel, act, and think like a rejuvenated and reinvented person!

Everything changes into a new YOU!

It is only through engaging with aromatherapy that you can achieve such a total transformation. After all, the regimen manages almost all the known health issues precipitated by inflammation that affect most people nowadays.

This book has guided you comprehensively to the ways and byways of your aromatherapy journey. Just remember that artificial fragrance can be toxic. Be true to yourself. Have the honor to surround your being with only the most organic and the purest possible aromatics, including all personal care items and household cleaning products.

At this point, you have certainly accomplished the mission of gaining the inspiration and information that you need to make aromatherapy a lifestyle- your new way of life. As to your response and direction, a new challenge faces you through this book's encouragements:

The next step is to encourage you now to make informed and mindful decisions about how to celebrate the joys of aromatherapy and use it in its best ways possible.

Embrace the social responsibility of spreading your eventual success: recipes, tips, techniques, positive testimonials, etc. Share your joys with everybody. Use and diffuse your essential goodness as your soulmate does in constant effectiveness to heal and help others!

Made in the USA
Las Vegas, NV
23 February 2024